HAND MUDRAS

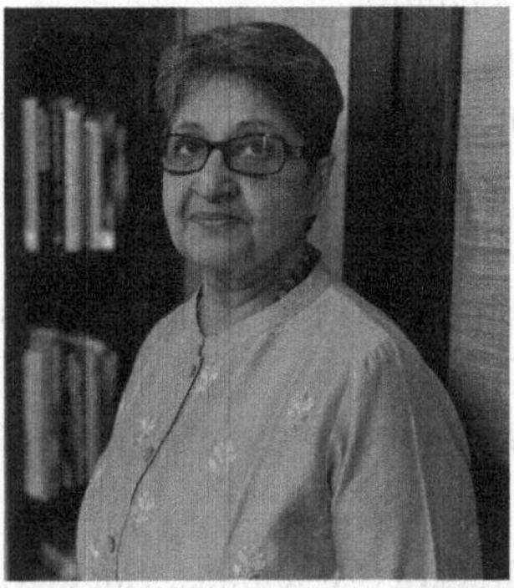

Premlata Haralalka is a renowned spiritual teacher and mudra healing expert who has dedicated the last three decades of her life to spreading the transformative power of ancient wellness practices. After retiring from a successful career as a travel entrepreneur twenty-five years ago, she embarked on a full-time spiritual mission to make mindful living accessible to people worldwide.

Trained under the guidance of Reiki Grandmaster Baba Sri Sri Muralidharan, Premlata has become a leading voice on hand mudras, Reiki and meditation. Her deep understanding of the Vedas and Upanishads guides her approach to integrating ancient wisdom with modern wellness requirements.

She has personally trained more than 50,000 students globally on the benefits of mindful living practices. Her teaching methodology—which breaks down complex spiritual concepts into practical, everyday applications—has earned her recognition across multiple wellness platforms and communities. She continues her mission through workshops, online courses and partnerships with leading wellness organisations.

To learn more about her transformative work, visit www.mudraswithprem.com.

'Over 45,000 Habuild members have benefited from our 5-day hand mudra workshop—a collaboration that began in 2023 with the renowned Dr Premlata. Since then, we have organised the workshop twice a year, offering our members the opportunity to explore the profound impact of mudras on their well-being.

The results have been inspiring! Many members have shared how mudra practices have improved their daily lives. One remarkable story comes from a member who, when faced with a broken elevator, used Apana Mudra to effortlessly climb four to five flights of stairs! This is just one of many examples of how these simple yet powerful practices are making a real difference.

Life-enhancing practices such as hand mudras have brought a positive difference to our community.'

—**Saurabh Bothra** (*Co-founder, Habuild*)

'Truly enriching experience. It provided great insights about mudras and their impact on energy, focus and well-being. The content was well-structured, making it easy to follow even for someone new to the practice. One of the best aspects was the wide range of topics covered. Premlata is a wonderful trainer.'

—**Tanushri Pal Chowdhury** (*Leadership Coach, Breathwork Facilitator and Spinal Energetics Practitioner, Netherlands*)

'Every session of this 5-day advanced mudra course was both very informative and enlightening, covering everything from inner and outer Chakra Mudras to Gayatri Mudras. I highly recommend this advanced course to everyone after completing the basic course. Premji is an excellent teacher; she explained even complex hand mudras very easily, while relating them to the divine knowledge of the Vedas, Upanishads and Patanjali's Yoga Sutras. It is an honor to have Premlataji as our mudra guru.'

—**Atul Batra** (*Product Management Executive, USA*)

'Thank you for an amazing journey; it came at the right time for me. All the mudras were demonstrated clearly, and the order in which they were explained was helpful. There was enough time to clear our doubts. I'm looking forward to joining the group and attending future classes.'

—**Geetha Anand** (*Researcher in Indian Philosophy, USA*)

'The course was extremely useful and well taught. The descriptions of each mudra's benefits and uses were informative and engaging, and the instructions were very clear and easy to follow. I received very useful tips which I have already started practising. So, a big thank you!'

—**Vaijayanti Bal** (*Founder, Aviation Charter Services, New Delhi*)

'Diagnosed with breast cancer and having undergone MRM surgery, I haven't had an easy time. I will soon begin chemotherapy. Throughout this period, I have drawn support from the regular practice of the mudras you recommended to maintain my well-being during cancer treatment. My sincere gratitude for your sessions. They have been invaluable, calming my mind and making me strong in this difficult phase of my life.'

—**Padmini Maurya**

'I had been suffering from severe knee pain for several days. During the advanced mudra course, Ma'am taught the Mooladhara Chakra Mudra. Practising this mudra for just five minutes over two days completely relieved me of my pain. I am thankful to Ma'am for sharing such a wonderful technique.'

—**Poonam Somaiya** (*Pranic Healer and Access Consciousness Practitioner*)

'My father was dealing with extremely dry skin, and no lotions or creams offered relief. Practising Jala Mudra completely resolved the problem. Additionally, Merudananda Mudra followed by Prana Mudra has significantly reduced his lower back pain.'

—**Nivedita Aradhey** (*Yoga Therapist and Pranic Healer*)

'Currently, we are in Texas, where pollen levels are high. My husband suffers from severe allergies, and both Linga Mudra and Aditi Mudra have been doing him wonders. Also, Apana Vayu Mudra has helped with his lower back pains. I am fascinated by the spiritual side of mudras, and when I attended your course and saw you perform the Gayatri Mudra, I was simply mesmerised. I am grateful for the opportunity and committed to applying myself seriously to the practice.'

—**Lalitha Sreenivasan** (*Trainer Educator – Hearfulness Meditation*)

'My mother, aged 83, had been suffering from chronic constipation for years. Suchi Mudra has turned out to be a saviour during this difficult time. Additionally, Bronchial Mudra and Kubera Mudra have provided her relief from chronic asthma and sinusitis. The results she has experienced through these mudras are amazing.

I have been hypertensive for the past three decades, and medicines did not resolve the issue. However, just a few minutes of daily practice of Kanishta Mudra has helped bring my blood pressure back to normal.

I am grateful to the Almighty for connecting me to hand mudras through Ma'am's teachings.'

—**Sharada M.R.** (*Retired Officer, LIC, Bengaluru*)

HAND MUDRAS

Transformative Yoga for Health and Wellness

PREMLATA HARALALKA

Published by Westland Books, a division of Nasadiya Technologies Private Limited, in 2025

No. 269/2B, First Floor, 'Irai Arul', Vimalraj Street, Nethaji Nagar, Alapakkam Main Road, Maduravoyal, Chennai 600095

Westland and the Westland logo are the trademarks of Nasadiya Technologies Private Limited, or its affiliates.

ISBN: 9789371979054

10 9 8 7 6 5 4 3

Hand mudra illustrations by R. Krishnan

Typeset by Jojy Philip

Printed at Manipal Technologies Limited, Manipal

ॐ

गुरुर्ब्रह्मा गुरुर्विष्णुः गुरुर्देवो महेश्वरः ।
गुरुः साक्षात् परं ब्रह्म तस्मै श्रीगुरवे नमः ॥

Gurur Brahmā Gurur Viṣṇuḥ Gurur Devo Maheśvaraḥ,
Guruḥ Sākṣāt Paraṁ Brahma Tasmai Śrī-Gurave Namaḥ.

With the deepest reverence and love, I dedicate this book to my revered guru Shri Muralidharan-ji and guruma Suseela-ji.

I bow at the lotus feet of Sri Baba and guruma, whose divine presence has been a constant source of inspiration and grace throughout the three decades of my spiritual journey.

Sri Baba's gentle yet powerful guidance—his silent teachings, his insistence on perfection in every action and his ability to convey the highest spiritual truths in the simplest of words—has been a shining beacon in my life.

The fruition of this book is nothing but a reflection of the unceasing kataksham that I continue to receive from Sri Baba. It is to his divine will and blessings that I offer this humble work.

Idam Na Mama

Contents

Specific Mudras

Foreword

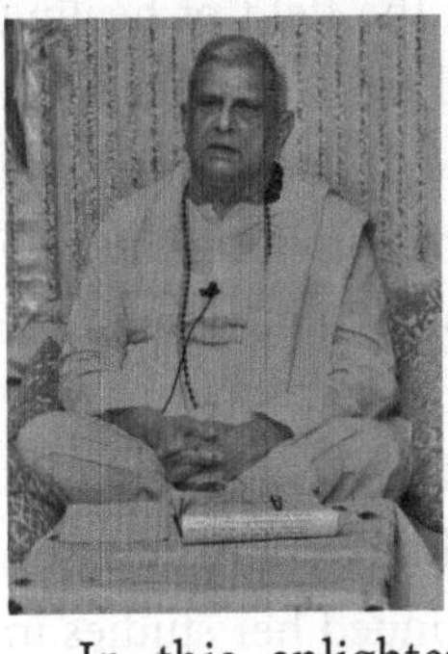

Throughout history, the quest for holistic well-being and spiritual awakening has guided countless seekers on a path of self-discovery. Among the many ancient techniques preserved through generations, mudras—powerful symbolic hand gestures—offer a unique and accessible avenue for healing the body and mind.

In this enlightening work, *Hand Mudras: Transformative Yoga for Health and Wellness*, we explore the profound healing potential of these sacred gestures. Rooted in ancient yogic wisdom, mudras are more than mere hand signs; they are tools to balance energies, restore vitality and cultivate mental clarity. Their simple yet potent nature allows anyone to integrate them into daily life, fostering physical health, emotional stability and peace of mind.

Whether you seek to alleviate specific ailments, reduce stress or cultivate inner harmony, this book provides practical insights and guided techniques to unlock the healing power within. By incorporating mudras into your routine, you can experience a wonderful transformation that nurtures both your body and mind.

It brings me great joy and reverence to introduce this illuminating work by Smt. Premlata. She has conducted thorough research on mudras from various authentic scriptures and compiled them effectively to provide comprehensive information to the reader, enhancing their ability to apply the knowledge competently. The illustrations, examples, explanations and instructions are presented systematically, making them easy for anyone to follow and practise.

This book on hand mudras is more than just a collection of gestures; it is a significant body of work in the field of healing sciences and arts. Premlata has approached this sacred subject with purity of intention and clarity of purpose. In these pages, she gently guides the reader towards inner balance, inviting them to experience the transformative power that resides quite literally in their own hands.

It was about twenty-five years ago that I met Smt. Premlata at one of my basic Reiki (Usui Natural Healing System) classes, among about eighty students. She then continued her studies in the Reiki healing system under my guidance until she reached the master's level. The master's level of initiation is reserved only for those who serve humanity with sincerity and dedication. I found in her all the qualities required to be initiated into the master's level. The journey of togetherness as guru and disciple began from then on, encompassing training and practice in meditation, past-life regression, various mental healing methods, Vedantic studies, and attending almost all satsangs on spiritual discourses. She showed great interest and devoted herself to all activities connected to these. Premlata has also transcribed my spiritual discourses and Vedic classes into books and published them. She has always wanted to be engaged in a service-oriented activity for the benefit of humanity; perhaps she discovered it through teaching the vidya of self-healing using mudras. A good-natured, gentle and soft-spoken person, as well as hardworking and dedicated in what she does, Premlata has earned great acceptance among her students.

May this work serve as a companion to those who seek health and harmony within. And may it inspire many to look inward with reverence and discover the sacred wisdom that has been passed down through the ages.

I wish Smt. Premlata all the best, and may God bless her with the ability to continue this good work for the benefit of humanity.

With blessings,
Swamy Muralidharan
30 June 2025
Kolkata

Preface

I have been actively involved in the spiritual learning, teaching and practising of Vedanta philosophy for over twenty-five years. When I completed my Reiki Level 1, my guru Sri Muralidharan-ji introduced me to the concept of the five elements and their connection to the fingers and hand positions. However, despite his demonstrations and chart-aided explanations, I did not take it seriously at the time.

As my spiritual practices deepened, especially through meditation, I was taught to hold the Bhairava Mudra and the Jnana Mudra. Over time, I discovered that the Bhairava Mudra naturally led me into a meditative state, while the Jnana Mudra brought a profound sense of calm. In just a few minutes, I would feel as though I wasn't even breathing—my mind would become completely still and peaceful!

This continued for a while, but I was still somewhat detached from the practice of mudras, and hence did not make the effort to study the subject extensively. It was about five years ago that my interest was truly rekindled and I began to dig deeper—I purchased books, researched online and watched YouTube videos. I began experimenting with mudras myself, and that's when I truly realised their powerful impact. I had already experienced the benefits of two mudras, but this exploration took it to a much deeper level. It led to the realisation that hand mudras gave us the power to heal ourselves holistically, as had already been discovered and written in our own ancient texts.

As I continued to study and experiment, I began sharing small mudras with others—simple ones that were safe to practise. It was interesting to discover that mudras help relieve physical ailments, alleviate mental and emotional problems, and aid spiritual growth. However, it should be remembered that though they are generally harmless, one must be cautious, as there are contraindications for certain practices.

I also started looking for formal courses to further my knowledge, but it took me almost a year to find a suitable programme. In the initial stages, I did enrol for a course, even though it was rather too expensive, but then realised that despite the dedicated one-to-one mentoring, it lacked a structured curriculum. Besides, one of the instructors made the honest admission that I knew more about the subject than them. I finally withdrew from the course.

In my quest to learn and deepen my understanding, I reached out to several other teachers, but met nobody who seemed confident enough in their approach. I found some ashrams that offered mudra courses, but most were very basic. An acharya I spoke with over the phone was very honest—when I mentioned that I wanted to understand the scientific basis behind the mudras, he told me, 'I don't think I'll be able to fulfil the purpose you have for doing this course.'

He mentioned that he would simply be following a particular book. That wasn't enough for me. In my search for a qualified programme, I looked online and found courses, but they were incredibly expensive—some as high as $500, even those offered by Indian teachers. This pushed me to explore the subject on my own through reading the right literature on the topic. I started collecting books from the Bihar School of Yoga, which, while not fully focused on mudras, provided valuable insights into the subject. I also heard of Acharya Keshav Dev and acquired several of his books. However, reaching out to his ashram ended up being near impossible and I had to drop all plans in that direction.

I considered studying with an acharya in Hyderabad, but his classes were taught in Telugu. It wasn't until a year later that they offered a session in English, which I eventually attended, though it came after two to three years of my own independent study, experimentation and research. Given that it was taught by yoga teachers, the course didn't go in-depth into theory but it did give me a basic idea.

With a stack of books, online resources and scriptures at my disposal, I began to delve deeper, trying to crystallise exactly what I wanted to learn. Having spent significant time studying under my guru and self-publishing his books, I realised I needed to explore further. This led me to discover the wonderful connection of mudras with chakras and pancha pranas (the five prana vayus), and this helped shape my course of study.

When I first started offering my course, it was quite a challenging task to persuade people to join—it took six months before the programme attracted any significant interest. This was understandable because not many truly grasped the impact of the practice. Even with the availability of resources on YouTube and other platforms, convincing people about the value of mudras and the benefits of my curriculum required significant effort.

It felt like I had to push for enrolments, and at times I even offered classes for free. In fact, during my debut session, I invited a friend to attend at no cost. She called me immediately after the very first class. She said she was deeply moved and insisted on giving me a guru dakshina. The acknowledgement was incredibly encouraging.

Gradually, participants began experiencing real benefits, and this became a strong motivator for me. Participation grew organically as word-of-mouth spread positive reports about the classes.

I then remembered Habuild, an online yoga platform offering daily yoga lessons and various courses. Having been a member and beneficiary of the Habuild community, I reached out to them, proposing an awareness session. They were convinced and the event I conducted fetched excellent feedback. That moment was another significant breakthrough for me.

After six months, they contacted me again. Since the response had been phenomenal, they wanted to extend the session to a five-day course, to be offered thrice a year. They organised it twice in 2024, with more than 9,000 viewers watching live and the recorded version garnering over 20,000 viewers. I also started offering free awareness sessions through various organisations, including the Lions Club, Rotary Club, and a few specific platforms focusing on the health and wellness of senior citizens. Participants from these classes eventually ended up joining my intensive course—it was incredibly empowering to know that people were benefitting from hand mudras. In fact, a women's group approached me after attending one of my awareness sessions and requested a dedicated workshop in Hindi for a large group from their pan-India member base.

Once, I came across a YouTube video where two foreigners were discussing hand mudras. They were mispronouncing Jnana Mudra. The speaker was an Australian healer working on a PowerPoint presentation on the subject. I emailed her to correct the mistake, and she immediately responded, asking me to teach her the correct pronunciation. Later, she requested recordings of all the mudra names for her presentation, which I gladly provided. Knowledge attained is useless unless shared. I was glad to be of help to so many interested souls from across the world who share a passion for the subject.

In addition, a corporate organisation offered me the amazing opportunity to host an awareness session for their employees on International Yoga Day. During one of my sessions, a participant who runs a deemed university expressed interest in organising a workshop for all his employees as well.

After a few classes, participants began requesting recordings. Though hesitant at first, I eventually agreed. I was already sharing PDFs at the end of my sessions. Eventually, attendees wanted a ready reckoner, and so I developed a mudra guide to share with anyone who joined my sessions.

My journey of learning continues. I still research new mudras and consult with many people, and this has opened my eyes to the vast range of diseases and challenges people face. One of my most remarkable students is a seventy-year-old woman who, despite numerous ailments, including hearing loss, stammering and injuries, remained cheerful and eager. Her positive attitude was inspiring.

Over the years, as I conducted classes, I realised that people would benefit from incorporating these basic practices into their daily routine. Though simple, they can bring phenomenal changes. These small teachings have helped many people experience notable changes in their lives.

I always emphasise that mudras require dedication and faith. While some now believe you can practise them while walking, talking or even watching TV, I stress that for maximum benefit, focused meditation and concentration are essential. When practised with full attention, the benefits are intensified and come about more quickly.

One of the most rewarding moments in my journey of teaching came when a psychological counsellor from Dubai shared her experience. Despite reading several books and watching YouTube videos, she was quite confused about hand mudras until she attended my course. After the programme, she was fully convinced about the merits of mudras and planned to integrate them into her professional practice. This reaction was a major turning point for me.

It made me realise that no single book provided a comprehensive view of mudras; I had to read many to gather the necessary knowledge. I also found that my spiritual background spanning two decades was a blessing! This truly helped me understand the significance of my field of study, and connect science with spirituality.

In my course, I aim to provide a complete understanding of everything I have learnt, in a simple, user-friendly format. This is, again, the core intent behind writing this book—to compile information in one place and make it accessible to all. It will be presented in a narrative style, making the learning process more engaging.

A lot of the information in this book comes from what I have learnt from my guru, teachers and elders over the years. While I have drawn from various sources, some parts of my knowledge were passed down through oral teachings. Through this book, I aim to share my understanding of what I have been taught, what I have read and what I have experienced.

I have capitalised Sanskrit terms when they name specific mudras, tatvas, chakras, pranas or other formal systems. Generic and descriptive terms remain uncapitalised.

Come join me in diving into this intriguing, ancient, powerful practice for the betterment of our own well-being, and that of those around us. The key to our health and wellness lies in our own hands—quite literally.

CHAPTER 1

Introduction

OM SHRI GUROBHYOM NAMAHA

मुद्राभिः स्थिरतां देहे, मनसः शान्तिमेव च।
रोगान् नाशयते सर्वान्, मुद्रायोगं नमाम्यहम्॥

Mudrābhiḥ sthiratāṁ dehe, manasaḥ śāntimeva ca |
Rogān nāśayate sarvān, mudrāyogaṁ namāmyaham ||

Literally translated, the shloka states that mudras help attain stability in the body and peace of the mind. Our endeavour is to delve deeper and uncover the secrets of this science of healing.

In an era where modern medicine often comes with caveats—side-effects, unaffordable bills, unpredictable treatment periods and sometimes, unhappy results—many seek solace in the wisdom of ancient healing systems. Rooted in the Vedas and other age-old traditions, these holistic approaches offer profound insights into the nature of wellness, focusing on the fundamental principles of energy.

Throughout history, systems such as Ayurveda, yoga and traditional Chinese medicine have recognised the vital role of energy in maintaining health and harmony within the body, mind and spirit. Practices like sparsha chikitsa, Reiki, marma healing and chakra cleansing have long been recognised for their ability to restore balance and vitality by working directly with the body's energy pathways.

Today, as science digs further into the mysteries of the universe, it acknowledges what sages and healers have known for millennia: everything in the manifest universe is composed of packets of energy. From the tiniest subatomic particles to the vast expanse of the cosmos, energy permeates every aspect of our reality, including our own bodies. It exists in everything and everything exists in it.

Energy healing, once regarded with scepticism, is now gaining recognition as a valid means of promoting wellness and facilitating health recovery. By harnessing the innate intelligence of the body and tapping into its natural ability to mend itself, we can unlock profound healing potential. The science of hand mudras is a powerful healing approach that brings about holistic transformation.

HISTORY AND ORIGIN OF HAND MUDRAS

There is no definitive data on when and how mudras originated, although there is evidence that they have been used across the world since ancient times. People of all religions—and even those with no religious affiliation—have been practising them. In fact, mudras are natural to the body; we often see people sitting in different hand positions instinctively.

Throughout history, various cultures have recognised the significance of hand gestures in communication, healing and spirituality. In India, the practice of mudras dates back thousands of years, deeply rooted in the teachings of yoga, Ayurveda and meditation. These subtle yet powerful gestures are believed to channel energy flow, stimulate different parts of the brain, and evoke specific emotional and mental states. In fact, a paradigm shift is taking place in the world now, with scientists and researchers alike recognising the role that energy plays in healing.

Mudra vijnana (the science of mudras) is a relatively less explored aspect of the time-honoured discipline of yoga. Hand mudras, one of the energy healing systems, have been mentioned in many of the ancient scriptures. For instance, the *Shiva Samhita* describes mudras as essential practices for purifying the nadis (energy channels) and balancing the flow of prana (life-force) within the body. The *Gheranda Samhita* contains detailed instructions on various mudras, including hand mudras, as tools for awakening Kundalini energy and achieving heightened states of awareness. The *Hatha Yoga Pradipika* has descriptions of numerous mudras, among them those performed with the hands, to regulate the flow of energy within the body and facilitate meditation. Documentation of mudras can also be found in the *Mantra Shashtra*, *Upasana Shashtra* and *Nritya Shashtra*. The practice of mudras is widely embraced by saints and yogis across India, and by Buddhist monks in Tibet and Japan. Their use is also prominent in Bhutan, Myanmar and Indonesia.

The story of Matsyendranath gives us insight into the mythical origin of mudras. It is widely believed that he was born under an inauspicious star, which led his parents to throw him into the ocean, where he lived for twelve years in the belly of a fish. The fish swam to the banks and overheard Adiyogi Bhagavan Shiva imparting secret knowledge to Mata Parvati. In the *Gheranda Samhita* (3.4–5), Bhagavan says:

मुद्राणां पटलं देवि कथितं तव सन्निधौ ।
येन विज्ञातमात्रेण सर्वसिद्धिः प्रजायते ॥ 4 ॥
गोपनीयं प्रयत्नेन न देयं यस्य कस्यचित् ।
प्रीतिदं योगिनाञ्चैव दुर्लभं मरुतामपि ॥ 5 ॥

mudrāṇām paṭalaṃ devi kathitaṃ tava sannidhau |
yena vijñātamātreṇa sarvasiddhi: prajāyate || 4 ||
gopanīyaṃ prayatnena na deyaṃ yasya kasyacit |
prītidaṃ yogināñcaiva durlabhaṃ marutāmapi || 5 ||

Bhagavan Shiva explains that by merely possessing knowledge about the mudras, one attains sarva siddhi (all-pervading success). He emphasises the importance of practising these daily to attain peace and happiness, adding that this wisdom is not easily available, even to the gods. This heightens the significance of mudras. Bhagavan Shiva then requests Mata Parvati to keep this knowledge a secret—to be taught with discretion only to the deserving and dedicated; others, he says, are not eligible. Due to the secrecy involved—since mudras bestow infinite powers upon the practitioner—much of the knowledge about the science of mudras ended up being lost over time.

After twelve years of yoga sadhana in the belly of the fish, Matsyendranath (as he later came to be known) emerged as a siddha and was blessed by Bhagavan Shiva to spread this knowledge among humans. The Nath sampradaya is born from this lineage.

The word mudra comes from the root words mud, meaning happiness, and dravya, meaning to receive or draw forth; therefore, mudra means to receive happiness. मुदम् आनन्दम् ददती इति मुद्राः—Bhagavan Shiva says to Mata Parvati that the gods are pleased with the mudras. Essentially, they are a way of life that reflects divine qualities. Mudra also means a seal or a lock, and mudras lock the energy within the body. In the *Gheranda Samhita* (3.4), Maharishi Gheranda states: *mudraya sthirata chaiva*—mudras help in attaining steadiness; they help maintain a stable body and mind. According to the *Hatha Yoga Pradipika* and several other yogic texts, mudras are considered to be yoganga—an independent limb (branch) of yoga. Mudras are also seen as higher practices that lead to the activation of the pranas and chakras and, with regular execution, enhance psychic powers.

Healthy energy radiates from people who are physically and mentally well, and this transforms their own individual aura. Just as negative energy can be felt around those who are unwell, sound health emits positive energy. When it comes to physical health, miraculous benefits are available in mudra vijnana. Mudras that show effectiveness immediately may act as primary treatment and according to Acharya Keshav Dev, known for popularising mudra vijnana, they are akin to first aid.

SCIENTIFIC RESEARCH ON HAND MUDRAS

The human body is a miracle that no scientist has been able to replicate, and the human hand is the most perfect instrument created by nature. The hand performs numerous functions, all controlled by the brain. The tiny muscles in the hands have motor-neural endings which are responsible for executing movements that are precise, controlled and complicated. Our fingers, like the rest of our body, generate an electromagnetic field. The fingertips are constantly emitting a small electric current and subtle electromagnetic waves. They can hold many different shapes and forms, known as mudras, and these mudras work and heal at the physical, mental, emotional and spiritual levels of a person.

Placing your hands and fingers in different positions affects your brain. A mudra is a precise and scientific yogic function which helps develop your internal and external disposition in different ways. Mudras not only affect the one who forms them but can also potentially influence those who observe them in the process.

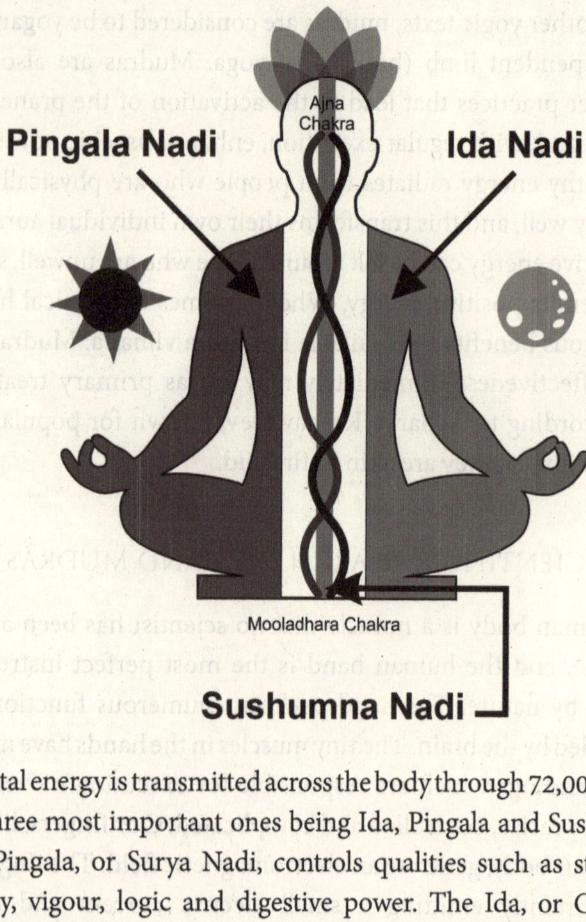

Vital energy is transmitted across the body through 72,000 nadis, the three most important ones being Ida, Pingala and Sushumna. The Pingala, or Surya Nadi, controls qualities such as strength, vitality, vigour, logic and digestive power. The Ida, or Chandra Nadi, controls feelings like appreciation, affection and tranquility, and governs our senses of taste and touch. It also determines creativity, and the health of a person's stomach and heart.

Vital energy from the cosmos enters the body through the Brahmarandhra and is emitted through the fingers and the surface of the body. It has no form and is invisible to the human eyes, but kirlian cameras can capture it. This vital energy, subtle in nature, is known as prana. The human body is continuously receiving and transmitting energy, and we can lock it into any particular channel as we desire. We may not be conscious of its flow within us, but it is active all the time—even as you read this. If we focus on it, we might even be able to feel the subtle energy.

MUDRAS AND THE BRAIN

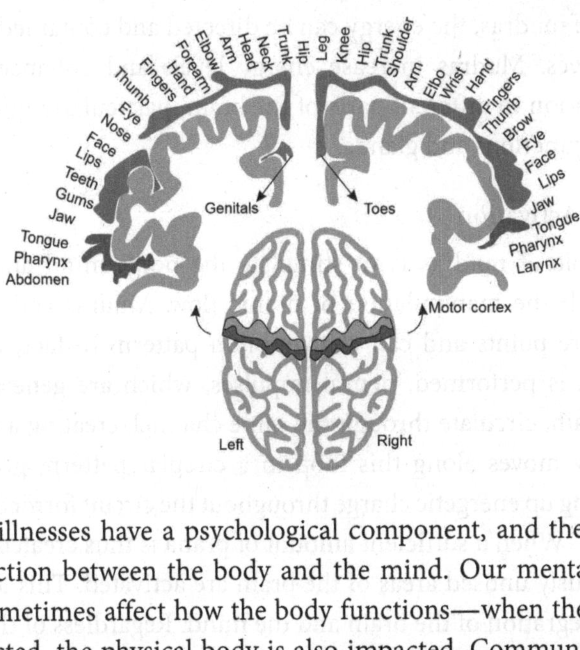

Some illnesses have a psychological component, and there is a connection between the body and the mind. Our mental state can sometimes affect how the body functions—when the mind is affected, the physical body is also impacted. Communication between the body and mind primarily occurs through the central nervous system, which consists of the spinal cord and the brain. Each hand has up to 1,00,000 nerve endings, with each finger having about 3,000 nerve receptors just under the skin's surface. The hands thus occupy a significant portion of the brain cortex, and each area of the hand is linked to a different part of the brain, as shown in the image.

WHAT DO HAND MUDRAS DO?

Nerve Connection

Hand mudras create an important connection in the nervous system and stimulate specific nadis. The nadis and chakras constantly emit prana—which we are typically not aware of—and this usually just dissipates into the atmosphere. With the help of mudras, the energy can be directed and contained within ourselves. Mudras increase energy levels and enhance blood circulation to different parts of the brain, particularly important nerve junctions and glands.

Brain Activation

The role of mudras is to stimulate the body, mind and brain through the manipulation of pranic flow. Mudras activate the pressure points and can change brain pattern. In fact, when a mudra is performed, neural impulses, which are generated in the brain, circulate through the same channel, creating a circuit. Energy moves along this loop in a circular pattern, gradually building up energetic charge throughout the circuit formed by the mudra. When a sufficient amount of prana is thus created, some previously unused areas of the brain are activated. This leads to the integration of the brain and the mind. Regardless of the kind of stimulation, whenever any mudra is performed, certain areas of the brain experience activity.

Transformation

As one continues practising mudras, regions of the brain that were previously dormant become progressively active in a process that is both harmonious and controlled. This can bring about many positive changes— for instance, certain fears, phobias, and mental or emotional problems may surface and dissolve. This means the negative charge stored in the corresponding brain area is released and the power of buddhi (intellect) increases. The negative charge is replaced with habits and patterns of thinking that are both creative and positive; in short, our behaviour undergoes a change, thereby leading to transformation.

HAND MUDRAS AND HEALTH

Cardiovascular Health

Several studies have investigated the effects of hand mudras on health parameters. The application of the Apana Vayu Mudra on heart patients revealed a substantial reduction in systolic and diastolic blood pressure, heart rate and blood viscosity. This study, conducted by Tripathi et al. (2017) proposes that the particular mudra makes its effect through the nerve endings in fingers. The mudra has a systemic effect on the cardiovascular system and improves it. The study reports that a doctor used this mudra on three patients suffering from severe chest pain. All three were stabilised and could then be safely transferred to the hospital for further treatment. Acharya Keshav Dev also supports the finding that this mudra is an on-the-spot supportive emergency tool for heart care.

Cognitive Function

Hand mudras are known to improve cognitive performance, including attention and memory, when performed regularly.

A study by Saraswat and Kumar (2021) confirms that regular practice of Jnana Mudra in normal, healthy people creates and improves mental toughness, while reducing levels of anxiety.

Posture and Pain Relief

Dentists assume stressful body postures which are necessary in their profession, but these stances often lead to musculoskeletal disorders. This is what prompted dentists like Dr Nitin Priyanka to resort to hand mudras that not only relieve pain but also help improve the overall well-being of the person. Even though Nitin et al. (2019) could not find scientific proof, solely based on their experience, they recommend certain mudras to be performed daily to remain pain-free and energetic.

Respiratory Health

The effect of lung-specific mudras on asthma patients was measured after six weeks of mudra practice. The mudras used were Pranamam Mudra, Bronchial Mudra, Asthma Mudra, Bhramara Mudra and Linga Mudra. The peak expiratory flow rate (PEFR), breath-holding time (BHT), Snider's test (ST), expiratory blast test (EBT) and respiratory endurance test (RET) were measured by Saravanan et al. (2019). This study concluded that lung-specific mudras improved lung-efficiency after six weeks of regular repetition. It also found that consistent practice of mudras could reduce the need for medication.

BENEFITS OF HAND MUDRAS

According to Acharya Keshav Dev, our ancient scholars have engaged in phenomenal research and experiments on hand mudras, and what we currently make use of is only a miniscule portion of their studies and knowledge.

Effective Therapy

- ☞ Mudras may be used to supplement conventional treatments for various ailments.
- ☞ They are non-invasive, have no side effects and can be safely used by anyone. They may appear simple, but the results can be surprising.
- ☞ Mudras need devoted practice to bring about changes in the human system. They affect the glands, nerves and energy channels. They help develop the internal and external disposition in different ways.

Balance of Energy

- ☞ Hand mudras facilitate healing, balance energy levels and keep the mind focused. In some cases, they can even bring about reversal of damage done to the human body and mind.
- ☞ Mudras help redirect and lock prana when necessary; they can awaken the inactive nerve cells and glands within us.

Mental Stability

- ☞ Mental stability, inner purification and recognition of the divinity within are some vital benefits of mudras, and these can be experienced by any regular practitioner.
- ☞ Mudras can alter the state of our consciousness. While this can be considered a mystery, they continue to help people find better directions in life.

Rituals and Spirituality

- ☞ Mudras can help sadhakas develop altered states of consciousness through regular practice. The subtle powers that lie dormant within can be awakened. Certain mudras redirect the prana emitted by the hands back into the body.

- ☞ Different mudras are used in different rituals and forms of worship. Mudras are seals, and when we seal the energy within our body, we prevent the mind from wandering. The mind becomes internalised—it calms and is drawn away from external objects; pratyahara (withdrawal of the five senses) takes place.

Ashta Siddhis

- ☞ Mudras are great tools for inner awakening and the attainment of siddhi. According to the *Hatha Yoga Pradipika*, siddhi denotes perfection of mind. The word siddhi is derived from two Sanskrit words: sidh, which means to go, to attains one's desires or achieve success; and dhi, which means intellect. Therefore, siddhi refers to the movement of the intellect towards higher goals, or the process of mental illumination. Lord Hanuman is associated with the ashta (eight) siddhis and hand mudras help us attain these.
- ☞ These are the eight siddhis through which one's intellect progresses as the mind is trained:

Siddhi	*Literal Meaning*	*Spiritual Significance*
Anima	The ability to reduce one's size to that of an atom.	The ability to become humble, reduce ego and become nothing.
Mahima	The ability to grow large in size.	The ability to think large and expand the consciousness.
Garima	The ability to become heavy.	The ability to stay grounded, attain inner steadiness and become steadfast in one's principles.

Siddhi	*Literal Meaning*	*Spiritual Significance*
Laghima	The ability to become weightless.	The ability to become detached from worldly desires.
Prapti	The ability to obtain one's goals.	The ability to focus mental energies and accept only what is necessary.
Prakamya	The ability to overcome obstacles.	The ability to fulfil selfless desires and live without negativity.
Ishitva	The ability to gain control over the pancha tatvas (the five elements).	The ability to attain control over the mind and emotions, thereby gaining freedom. It teaches one how to respond instead of reacting.
Vashitva	The power to attract.	The ability to influence another person's mind through love and inner purity.

☞ Even though Lord Hanuman possessed these siddhis, he never allowed them to distract him from his devotion to Lord Rama. The attainment of these siddhis itself denotes mastery over one's mind and emotions. Hand mudras aid in inner awakening, and these siddhis are the additional benefits one acquires. These ashta siddhis highlight what we can achieve once the ego dissolves.

WHAT MUDRAS CANNOT DO

Not everyone may experience the expected benefits of mudras, and this can happen for several reasons. First, it requires daily practice as specified, and for chronic diseases, practitioners may continue for weeks or even months before observing changes, if any.

Secondly, sometimes our own thoughts and emotions hinder our healing. While we make efforts by way of medicines or different forms of healing, we all love to attract sympathy: constantly talking about the problems and mentally repeating the issues. In the process, we do not experience inner peace. Thus, while you perform hand mudras, your thoughts remain contradictory; hence, healing does not take place.

CLASSIFICATION OF MUDRAS BY TYPES

Though people usually associate the term yoga with only yogasanas, any action that leads to a union is yoga. Hence, mudras are a part of yoga. They connect different energies within the a person to different parts of the body; युज्यते इति मुद्रा: (yujyate iti mudrāhā)—That which unites is called a mudra.

Yoga mudras have been classified into several types:

- Hastha Mudras: involves the use of the palms and fingers to form gestures used for chikitsa, rituals and worship.
- Mana Mudras: involves the sense organs, like the Chakshu Mudras.
- Kaya Mudras: involves postural mudras that uses the complete body, like Bhujangini Mudra, Vipareet-Karani Mudra, etc.
- Adhara Mudras: involves the pelvic floor muscles, like the Ashwini Mudra.
- Bandha Mudras: involves bandhas like the Ujjayi Bandha, Moola Bandha and Jalandhara Bandha.

Hastha (hand) mudras can be further classified, and this book focuses specifically on this category.

MUDRAS: THREE STYLES OF HAND PLACEMENTS

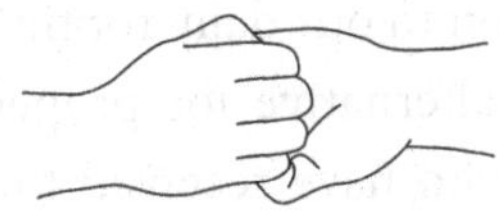

Joined hands: Pankaja Mudra, Pranamam Mudra, Ganesha Mudra, etc.

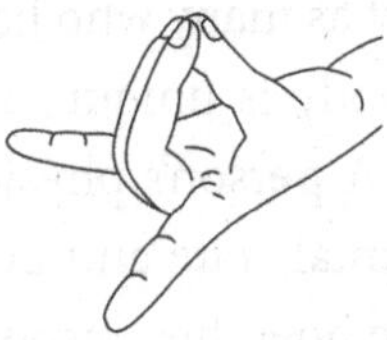

Separate hands (both hands in the same mudra): Apana Vayu Mudra, Jala Mudra, etc.

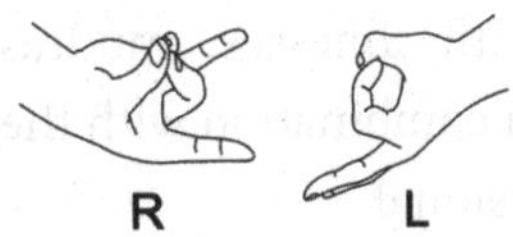

Dual mudras (each hand in a different mudra): Kati Mudra, Bhramari Mudra, Keela Mudra, etc.

* * *

Mudras can express feelings and sentiments, as in the case of Bharatanatyam mudras. We can see mudras being used by religious figures—Lord Buddha and Sri Gurunanak are seen in Abhaya Mudra while Jesus Christ is portrayed holding the Prana Mudra. We too, often unconsciously, sit holding certain hand mudras.

As we conclude this chapter, we have laid the foundation for understanding the profound impact that hand mudras can have on our physical and mental well-being. The upcoming chapters will delve deeper into the science behind pancha tatvas, chakras and pancha pranas, shedding light on how these interact within the human system. We will also explore a wide array of mudras, providing detailed guidance on hand formations and their specific benefits. By classifying these mudras into different categories, this book aims to make it easier for you to identify the most effective practices for various ailments and to harness the full potential of mudras in your daily life.

While mudras can be a valuable addition to our daily routine to promote well-being, they are not an alternative for proper medical treatment. For as many people who have received the benefits of mudra practice, there are likely just as many who have not experienced any effects. Every human body is unique, and the results can vary from person to person. A person's physical condition, their level of receptivity, their mental state and even their surrounding environment can influence how they respond to mudras. Therefore, when dealing with illnesses, mudras should be used as a supportive measure, in combination with the treatment suggested by a healthcare professional.

CHAPTER 2

Guidelines on Mudras

Mudras are simple hand gestures that can have profound effects. To get the best results, it's important that you follow the proper guidelines. Washing your hands before starting, sitting upright with a straight spine and deep breathing can all enhance the practice. At first glance, they might seem like minor details. However, they have a significant impact on our body, mind and energy. These elements are vital in allowing mudras to work effectively.

TIME AND DURATION

Mudras should generally be practised for at least fifteen minutes at a time, except when specified otherwise. The electromagnetic field is created in just thirty seconds. Those with no ailments should hold specified mudras for ten minutes each to maintain their health and well-being.

For therapeutic purposes, four to five mudras should be selected based on individual needs. Therapeutic mudras should not be performed immediately after meals. It is best to wait at least an hour after eating. These should be practised for a total of fifty minutes, split into three sessions, and most of these mudras take atleast forty-five minutes before any changes might be triggered in the body. Therapeutic mudras should be discontinued once the health issue is resolved.

Consistency is key. Practicing mudras at the same time each day can attune the body to the routine and increase effectiveness. Beginners should start with fewer mudras for shorter periods of time, gradually increasing the number and duration.

Mudra practice first releases negative charges, then builds positive ones. So do not expect overnight results. You will see changes, but they will be gradual.

POSTURE AND PLACE

Hand Position

Hand mudras are best done using both hands. Before you begin, rub your palms together till they become warm, as this enhances blood flow, which in turn makes energy flow smoother and more productive, boosting the effectiveness of the mudras. Unless specified, place your hands on your knees, palms up, while doing mudras. This helps energy flow through a hidden channel (Gupt Nadi) to your Mooladhara (Root) Chakra, waking it up and then moving up to your brain through the central energy path (Sushumna Nadi).

Lightly touch your fingertips together and straighten your other fingers. Initial difficulty may indicate bodily issues. You should be able to experience tingling between fingers but the contact should be light. This ensures that the energy flow is smooth and proper. The light touch is what helps maintain sensitivity and connection between fingers by enhancing the effect of the practice. Holding the mudra position precisely may be challenging at first—the fingers might slip or may not straighten at first, but with repetition, they will develop dexterity and the mudras will stabilise. However, mudra practice should be painless. If you experience pain when holding mudras, adjust the finger position. Ignoring the pain can lead to injuries.

Reiki practitioners can mentally draw symbols on their palms.

Ideal Posture

While some mudras have rules, most are simple. It is best to sit in a meditation pose when doing mudras. A straight spine enables the flow of energy along the spinal column. The most ideal way to practise is by sitting in the same place every day, facing east or north, in a comfortable meditative posture like Vajrasana or Padmasana. Clip your nails and wear loose, comfortable clothing. When sitting on a chair, use a mat under your feet to prevent loss of energy.

Be Mindful

The right mindset helps too. Do not hold mudras when in a bad mood or an unbalanced state of mind, except in emergencies. Your emotional state has a direct impact on the effectiveness of mudras.

You do not need to close your eyes while practising mudras, but it can help you notice small changes in your body and mind more easily. You might feel shifts in energy, breathing, body heat or emotions. Thus, body awareness is enhanced. Besides, concentration intensifies the effect of the mudras.

The body has its own intelligence, and gives us signals. Listen to your body's cues—if you feel any discomfort like dizziness or nausea, stop the mudra and try another one. Mudras should make you feel relaxed and at ease.

Mudras generate heat in the body, so it is important to drink plenty of water before and after mudras.

Flexibility

In today's fast-paced world, it may not always be practical to have a dedicated practice space. You can do mudras anywhere, anytime—sitting, standing, walking or even lying down. All that matters is that you are comfortable. However, spiritual mudras have to be performed in a meditative posture.

Mudras can be performed at any hour of the day but certain mudras that generate heat should not be performed during peak summers or at noon.

MINDFUL PRACTICE

Synchronised Breathing

Practise deep breathing several times before you start holding mudras, as it helps release the expended or stale energy accumulated within you. Smooth, calm breathing enhances benefits and stability, as the mind and body are completely relaxed. Synchronising mudras with breathing yields faster results, as it supports undivided attention and mindfulness. You experience the energy generation and flow within the body. Practising mudras with full focus and awareness can lead to profound changes in the body, mind and spirit. Working on your breath retention after every inhalation and exhalation can also enhance the power of mudras.

Combining Mudras

Mudras can be combined with any form of medical treatment to potentially accelerate the healing process. When applicable, chanting mantras while holding the mudras can bring about faster results.

* * *

Mudras can offer benefits when practised correctly. They can help balance the elements, energies and chakras in the body. Understanding concepts like pancha tatvas, chakras and pancha pranas can help identify the right mudras for healing.

CHAPTER 3

Pancha Tatvas and Mudra Vijnana

This chapter explores the concept of the five elements (pancha tatvas) and their connection to the human body, as well as the practice of mudra vijnana, a yogic technique for balancing these elements and promoting healing.

THE FIVE ELEMENTS IN THE HUMAN BODY

The human body, as per the *Garbhopanishad*, is composed of the same five elements as the cosmos—Earth (Prithvi Tatva), Water (Jala Tatva), Fire (Agni Tatva), Air (Vayu Tatva) and Space or Ether (Akasha Tatva). Earth provides solidity and structure, Water facilitates digestion and assimilation, Fire fuels dynamism, Air enables movement and Ether allows for expansion. These elements are interconnected and interdependent, and their balance is crucial for our health and well-being. They are not merely physical substances but rather energetic forces that govern various aspects of our being.

That the human body is made up of the same five elements as the universe can be observed when the physical form disintegrates. When the body perishes, it becomes cold, implying it can no longer retain heat (Fire); the body then bloats up (Air); then it decomposes with the help of its own liquid contents (Water); the remaining physical structure then breaks down and degrades into dust (Earth); and finally, it evaporates into air (Ether).

The slightest imbalance in the pancha tatvas can lead to diseases and difficulties. Mudras, through their manipulation of prana shakti, can help us direct this energy and restore balance. They enhance the power of intuition, promote mental stability and help us lead a stress-free life. Powers lying dormant within can be activated. The human body has the capacity to heal itself but we largely remain unaware of the potential we have. The schema of age-old practices and culture has influenced our way of thinking and emotions, hindering the healing process.

Science has made tremendous progress but many people across the globe are moving towards alternative methods of healing now. Our ancient seers perhaps knew what was to come and hence left a treasure trail for us to follow. With the help of yogic practices such as yogasanas, pranayama, meditation, sparsha chikitsa and mudra vijnana, we can tap into these powers and use them effectively.

THE FIVE ELEMENTS AND ANCIENT SCRIPTURES

The role and importance of the five elements are emphasised in many of our scriptures. The *Garbhopanishad* states that the five elements make up the human body, and along with it, the mind, intellect and ego shape the individual nature and human experience. In Chapter 7 of the Bhagavad Gita, Bhagavan Sri Krishna explains the relevance of the five elements to Arjuna. He says earth, water, fire, air, ether, mind, intellect and egoism are his eight-fold prakriti (nature):

भूमिरापोऽनलो वायु: खं मनो बुद्धिरेव च |
अहङ्कार इतीयं मे भिन्ना प्रकृतिरष्टधा || 7.4 ||

bhūmir-āpo ’nalo vāyuḥ khaṁ mano buddhir eva cha
ahankāra itīyaṁ me bhinnā prakṛitir aṣhṭadhā

In *Taittiriya Upanishad*, Bhagavan says that Akasha (Ether) was created from his material energy; from Akasha came Vayu (Air); from Vayu came Agni (Fire); from Agni, Apaha (Water); from Apaha, Prithvi (Earth); from Prithvi, food; and from food, man.

तस्माद्वा एतस्मादात्मन आकाशः सम्भूतः । आकाशाद्वायुः ।
वायोरग्निः । अग्नेरापः । अद्भ्यः पृथिवी ।
पृथिव्या ओषधयः । ओषधीभ्योन्नम् । अन्नात्पुरुषः । 2.1 ।

tasmādvā etasmādātmana ākāśaḥ sambhūtaḥ | ākāśādvāyuḥ |
vāyoragniḥ | agnerāpaḥ | adbhyaḥ pṛthivī |
pṛthivyā oṣadhayaḥ | oṣadhībhyonnam | annātpuruṣaḥ |

THE FIVE ELEMENTS AND THEIR TANMATRAS

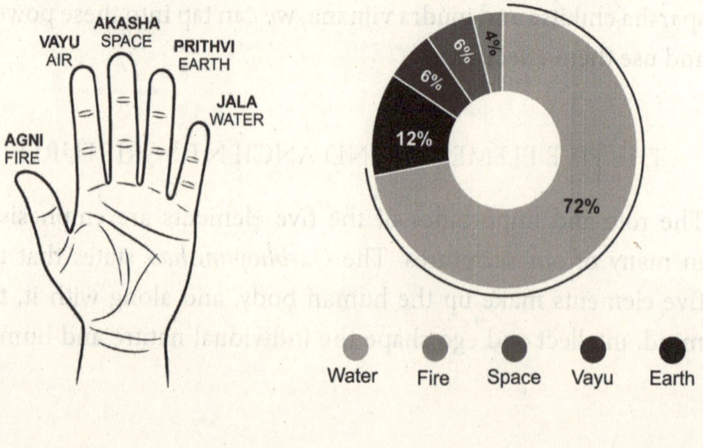

The human body is composed of five elements, with each finger representing an element. The little finger represents Water, which makes up 72 per cent of the body. The Fire element, represented by the thumb, comprises 4 per cent. The Air and Ether elements account for 6 per cent each and are represented by the index and middle fingers, respectively. The ring finger represents the Earth element, which makes up 12 per cent of the body's composition.

The five elements should not be mistaken for ordinary matter—for instance, the earth or water—we see around us. The consciousness is an energy that manifests itself in five elements—the pancha tatvas. These are pranic vibrations and they have a major influence on the mind and emotions. Each of the five fingers represent one element and by holding mudras as per requirement, we can balance the tatvas in the body. Every element has its own nature and characteristics, and governs different functions.

Each element also has an organ of perception (jnanendriya) and an organ of action (karmendriya) related to it. Before the five elements appear in their gross form, they exist in their pure form, known as tanmatra (each is alone, by itself). These subtle essences are the root energies from which the gross elements emerge. They are responsible for our sensory experiences and can influence our mind and emotions. Everything comes into creation because of tanmatras. An understanding of these will help us to ascertain which mudra is to be performed.

The five jnanendriyas are the ears, skin, eyes, tongue and nose. The corresponding tanmatra are shabda (needs space to travel), sparsha (experienced through skin), roopa (seen with the eyes), rasa (tasted using the tongue) and gandha (perceived through the nose).

Tatva	*Tanmatra*	*Related Organs*
Akasha Tatva—Space or Ether	Shabda (sound)	Sound can be heard through the element of Ether; the organs of hearing are the ears. The organ that generates sound is the mouth.
Vayu Tatva—Air element	Sparsha (touch)	Touch is the quality of Air and this sensing is possible through the skin.
Agni Tatva—Fire element	Roopa (form)	The quality of Fire is form and this can be perceived through the eyes.
Jala Tatva—Water element	Rasa (taste)	The quality of Water is taste and it is connected to the tongue.
Prithvi Tatva—Earth element	Gandha (smell)	The quality of Earth is smell and it is related to the nose.

INCREASING, DECREASING AND BALANCING TATVAS

An imbalance, whether one of excess or deficit of an element in the body, can lead to diseases. This means that the same element can either harm or heal us, depending on its proportional presence. Modern lifestyle changes have disrupted this balance, and as a result, people frequently experience stress, tension and mental health conditions. For instance, people often do not take the time to eat properly, resulting in disharmony of the elements in the body and potential diseases.

There are mudras that can help rectify this condition and aid in restoring the balance of elements in our body. For each tatva that is out of balance, there is a mudra that can restore it. We will be listing these in the following sections.

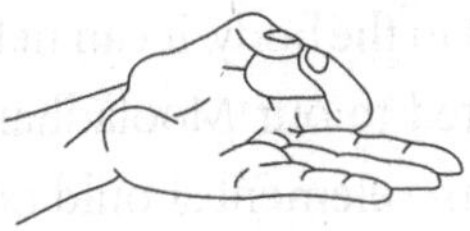

1. To balance the element: when we touch the tip of the thumb to the concerned element, the element's balance is restored.

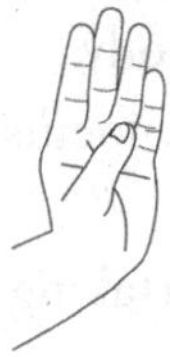

2. To increase the element: when we touch the pad of the thumb to the base of any finger, the corresponding element increases.

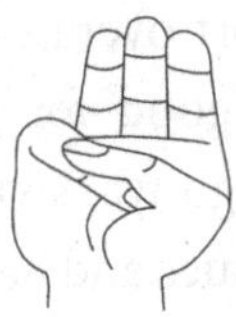

3. To decrease the element: when we press down on a finger using the thumb, the concerned tatva is decreased.

PRITHVI TATVA: EARTH ELEMENT

Prithvi Tatva represents Earth, the element that provides stability, solidity and strength. Its tanmatra is gandha. Prithvi Tatva governs the sturdiness of our bones, muscles and other organs. It gives vigour, form and structure to the body; it is considered responsible for weight and density. When this element is out of balance, one may experience fatigue, weakness, greed, loss of appetite or skin problems.

Hand Formation: Prithvi Mudra—associated with the ring finger (anamika)

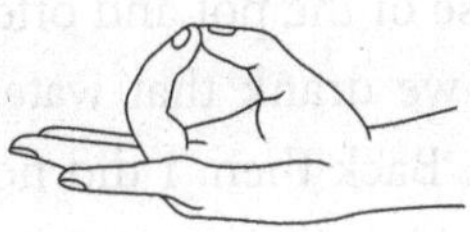

- Lightly touch the tips of the ring finger and thumb.
- Keep the other three fingers straight but relaxed.

Benefits:

- Restores equilibrium to the Earth element in the body. It can help rectify any deficiencies or illnesses related to our Mooladhara Chakra or the Earth element. However, the element should not be both increased and decreased on the same day.
- Leads to better pranic circulation within the body.
- During pregnancy, it is believed to help the foetus absorb proper nutrition.
- Holding the mudra for ten minutes before partaking in food can provide you with general health benefits.
- This mudra is generally practised to support overall health. There are anecdotal evidence of it being good for gastric ulcers, poor digestion, lack of smell, chikungunya, swine flu, weakness, dandruff, dehydration, urinary issues and hair loss.
- It helps ease negative thoughts.

JALA TATVA: WATER ELEMENT

Water possesses the quality to bind things together and, hence, is a constructive force. Jala Tatva represents Water, the element that governs fluidity, purification and nourishment. Its tanmatra is rasa. Jala Tatva controls the movement of energy and fluids in the physical body.

Water has memory, and the way we interact with it can influence its properties. Reflecting on my childhood, I now understand some of the practices I observed. I remember seeing water brought into the house in pitchers or mud pots, placed on the kitchen counter but not consumed immediately. My grandmother would light a lamp at the base of the pot and offer flowers. It wasn't until the next day that we drank that water. Two pots were always placed side by side. Back then, I did not understand why we did this.

As I grew spiritually, I began to understand the significance of these actions. In ancient times, especially during the Dwapara and Treta Yugas, nature was revered, and Water, being one of the five elements, was devoutly worshipped. Today, our water travels through pipes with many twists and turns, and its natural structure may get disrupted by the time it reaches us. Even after filtration, it is beneficial to let the water stand for a while so that it can regain its natural characteristics.

Another mindful way to consume water is to fill a cup or glass in the morning, hold it with both hands so that all ten fingers touch the glass, and gaze at it with reverence. Chant the Gayatri Mantra five, seven or eleven times while holding the water, and then drink it with the understanding that it is cleansing and purifying you. Vedic philosophy suggests that chanting mantras while observing water can alter its molecular structure.

In the body, the Water element appears as blood, saliva, tears, urine, sweat, semen and breast milk. Therefore, when the Jala Tatva is out of balance, it may lead to issues with digestion, excretion, menstrual flow and bladder control.

Hand Formation: Jala Mudra—associated with the little finger (kanishta)

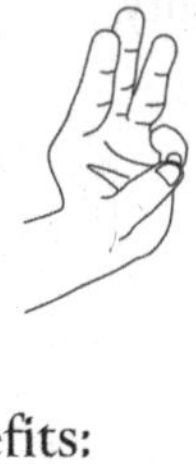

- Lightly touch the tips of the little finger and thumb.
- Keep the other three fingers upright and close to each other.

Benefits:

- The Jala Mudra can be effective for skin problems, and I have personally benefitted from it when I contracted herpes. I would hold this mudra for thirty minutes twice a day, and even the doctor was surprised when I mentioned that uncharacteristically, I did not experience any pain at all.

- Another instance was when I had a stomach infection and woke up with abrasions on my tongue, along with roughness on my lower gums and upper palate. I decided against consulting a doctor and instead focused on Jala Mudra. I would do it for about forty-five minutes during the day, spread out over two to three sittings. There was incremental improvement every day and it only took me approximately a week to recover.
- Jala Mudra is said to be effective for relieving dry eyes as well, particularly in people who work or live in an air-conditioned environment.
- After a course of antibiotics, it's common to find your taste buds affected, leaving food tasting bland and lacking flavour. The usual enjoyment of meals and your appetite can be diminished, as the palate temporarily loses its sense of taste. The Jala Mudra is believed to help correct the sense of taste.
- The mudra promotes kidney and bladder health.
- Practitioners have reported that it works equally well for cracked heels, dry mouth, dry cough and the purification of blood.
- It stimulates the salivary glands, which can help relieve thirst.
- The mudra fosters creativity and mental flexibility.

Contraindications:

- Should not be performed by those with edema.
- Should be paused during the menstrual cycle.

AGNI TATVA: FIRE ELEMENT

Movement of air creates friction, and friction creates fire. Agni Tatva represents Fire, the element that fuels dynamism, energy and willpower. Its tanmatra is roopa. Agni Tatva is responsible for digestion, the transformation of thoughts and the regulation of our internal heat.

Agni is the adhipati (lord) as it influences all the other elements. In fact, Agni Tatva is used to balance, increase or decrease any tatva as necessary. When the thumb touches another finger, the excess energy in that finger is drawn out by the thumb, and the equilibrium, or balance of energy, is restored.

Imbalance of this element can lead to lack of motivation and concentration, poor decision-making, problems with impulse control, and issues related to elimination and digestion. If the Earth element is high, it can destroy the Fire element. This can cause disharmony, leading to laziness, lethargy and heaviness. Surya Mudra stimulates the Fire element while also pacifying the Earth element.

Hand Formation: Surya Mudra—represented by the thumb (angushta)

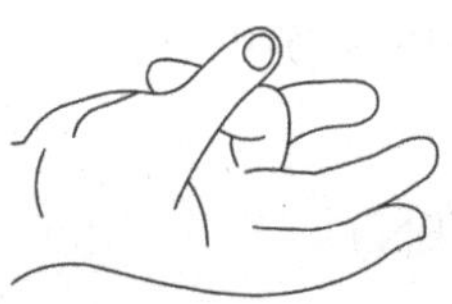

- Place the tip of the ring finger at the base of the thumb.
- Press the ring finger down with the thumb.
- Keep all the other fingers straight but relaxed.

Benefits:

- People with low metabolism are known to practise this mudra to reduce weight. However, it should not be blindly used to combat obesity or weight gain. The underlying reason for the condition needs to be identified first, as the Surya Mudra can cause hyperacidity and generate a lot of heat when used in the wrong situation.

- ☞ This mudra is often used to regulate digestion, appetite, thirst and sleep.
- ☞ Surya mudra is beneficial for the eyes.
- ☞ It is also useful in cases of sinusitis and headaches related to colds—but other specific mudras have been identified for these.
- ☞ The Surya Mudra helps purify the blood.

Contraindications:

- ☞ Those with low kapha constitution or high pitta constitution should practise the mudra in moderation, as it can lead to high acidity.
- ☞ Weak people should avoid this mudra as it can cause weight loss.
- ☞ Should not be performed by those with glaucoma.
- ☞ This mudra should not be practised for more than ten minutes at a stretch as it generates a lot of heat.
- ☞ It should not be done in peak summers.
- ☞ It may prove harmful to one's health unless plenty of water is consumed before and after the mudra is practised.

VAYU TATVA: AIR ELEMENT

Vayu Tatva represents Air, the element that governs movement and dynamism. Its tanmatra is sparsha. The skin is very sensitive and can easily detect changes in pressure or vibration at the subtle level. According to Ayurveda, several imbalances and illnesses may result from an excess of wind or air.

Hand Formation: Vayu Mudra—represented by the index finger (tarjani)

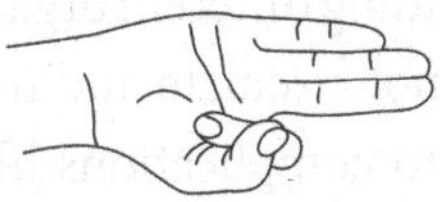

- Touch the tip of the index finger to the base of the thumb.
- Press the index finger down with the thumb.
- Keep all the other fingers straight but relaxed.

Benefits:

- Vayu Mudra helps release the excess air in the body. A patient once observed that after holding Vayu Mudra, he experienced uncharacteristic flatulence. This is because our body often contains excess air that needs to be released; this mudra helps with that. At times, we might not even be aware that the body contains excess vayu.
- The mudra can aid with gout, rheumatism, sciatica, hand tremors and headaches.
- The release of excess air in the body can help with bad posture, disturbed bodily functions, intestinal toxins, emotional problems and psychological issues. There are practitioners who have reported that this mudra has helped alleviate pains of all kinds—particularly back pain—and improve facial paralysis, arthritis, excess vata, imbalanced pitta, excessive anger, sleep issues and stress. The mudra can be practised for up to fifty minutes in a day, spread out over as many as three sittings.

AKASHA TATVA: SPACE OR ETHER

Whenever the word akasha is uttered, the mind visualises an open space or vastness. Akasha Tatva represents Space, or Ether, the element that provides the scope for matter to exist. Its tanmatra is shabda. Sound is perceived by the ears.

Akasha Tatva is the subtlest of the five elements—all-pervading and motionless. It controls the space surrounding different organs in the human body. Without space, air cannot circulate and this can create congestion in the heart or lead to complications like paralysis, choking, heart issues and suffocation.

Sound is generated when the vocal cords vibrate. Hence, any disease concerning the ears, larynx, vocal cords or throat is associated with the Akasha Tatva. This tatva governs communication, speech, intuition, dreams, clairvoyance and spiritual consciousness. It is also responsible for all the gross, subtle and causal sound perceptions conveyed through the ears. Many diseases and illnesses, especially those connected to the ears, may occur due to imbalance of the Akasha Tatva.

As a child, I would often notice my grandparents performing a curious gesture whenever they yawned—lightly snapping their middle finger and thumb together. To my young mind, it appeared to be nothing more than an unconscious habit, a quaint peculiarity.

Only much later did I come to understand the quiet wisdom behind this act. What seemed casual was, in fact, a mindful practice deeply rooted in ancient tradition. By pressing the middle finger against the thumb—forming the sacred Akasha Mudra—they were consciously harmonising the subtle Ether element within their bodies. More practically, this simple mudra served to prevent the risk of the jaw locking—a vulnerability that increases with age.

In the quiet dignity of their movements, my grandparents embodied a profound truth: that life's smallest actions, when performed with awareness, become sacred. Even something as ordinary as a yawn was met with mindfulness, respect for the body, and a deep alignment with nature's rhythms.

These gentle practices, passed down through generations, remind us that true wisdom often lies hidden in the simplest gestures, waiting patiently to be rediscovered.

Hand Formation: Akasha Mudra—represented by the middle finger (madhyama)

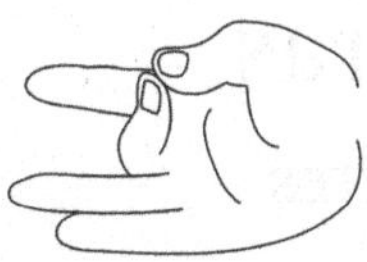

- Lightly touch the tips of the middle finger and thumb.
- Keep all the other fingers straight but relaxed.

Benefits:

- There are reports of the mudra relieving lockjaws.
- Users of the mudra mention that it helps with earaches and ear blocks—particularly caused by air travel. The mudra is also stated to aid in recovery from jet lag.
- When this element is in balance, one feels secure, connected, protected, loved and accepted.

* * *

For a healthy body and mind, it is essential to maintain a balance of these five elements. Besides, a balance is also a prerequisite for spiritual development. Disturbances in the physical body and mind occur when the equilibrium of the five elemental forces in the body is disturbed. Mudras are one of the methods used to restore or maintain the balance disrupted due to emotional upheavals. Consequently, healing takes place when stability is restored.

CHAPTER 4

Nadis and Chakras

A Guide to Energy Centres

This chapter explores the intricate network of nadis and chakras, vital energy centres within the human body. It delves into their significance in ancient yogic texts, their association with physical and mental well-being, and their role in spiritual awakening. We will examine the seven major chakras, their characteristics and how imbalances can manifest in our lives.

THE NADIS AND CHAKRAS: A COMPLEX SYSTEM

Scriptures like *Hatha Yoga Pradipika* and *Goraksha Samhita* state that the human body has 72,000 nadis (astral nerve tubes or energy channels) that transmit prana throughout the entire system. The number of nadis vary across texts. According to *Shiva Samhita*, there are 3,50,000 nadis but the hathayogis later simplified the system and reduced it to 72,000. Thus, we have 36,000 nadis on each side.

Nadis have no physical form. Prana vayu flows through the nadis, and wherever they intersect, there is a chakra. However, not all of these nadis cross each other. There is only one point at which they all converge—the Manipura Chakra, which is the vital energy centre that empowers our survival; without its strength and energy, nothing can be accomplished. The tatva in this chakra is Agni, which conforms to Agni being the adhipati as specified in the previous chapter. This chakra is considered the connection point between the foetus and the mother via the umbilical cord. To grasp these concepts, it is imperative that we understand chakras.

CHAKRAS: PSYCHIC CENTRES OF CONSCIOUSNESS

Chakras are psychic centres of consciousness, first mentioned in the *Yoga Upanishads* (600 BC) and later in the *Yoga Sutras of Patanjali* (200 BC). *Yoga Upanishads* is a collection of minor Upanishads including *Shandilya*, *Jabala*, *Chudamani*, *Teja Bindu* and *Yogashikha*.

Sri Aurobindo (2000) defines chakras as conscious centres and sources of all dynamic powers of our being, organising their actions through the plexuses and arranged in an ascending series from the lowest physical to the highest mental centre. This definition is based on his study of the system of chakras as understood in tantric knowledge and accepted in various yogic systems.

Ancient scholars have long emphasised the interconnectedness of physical, mental and spiritual health in human beings, a connection facilitated by the body's chakras. The word chakra in Sanskrit means wheel or vortex, reflecting their nature as spinning cosmic energy centres. These vortices, where matter meets life-force, or prana, are visualised as circular energy fields that exist within our subtle etheric body, though they have no physical form. Scientifically, they are often referred to as glandular junctions.

The seven major chakras in the body correspond to significant nerve centres and major glands. Although these chakras are located along the spine, they are easier to identify and visualise from the front. These energy centres absorb and distribute prana throughout the body, ensuring that it reaches all the organs. The lower five chakras are aligned from the base of the spine to the throat. Beyond the Throat chakra, the remaining two energy centres are located in the brain.

The human body contains three primary energy channels: the Sushumna in the centre, Ida on the left, and Pingala on the right. The chakras are located at the intersection of these three energy channels, where they spin prana shakti, or life energy, and distribute it to various organs.

For optimal health, the chakras must be aligned, energised and balanced. Disturbances can block the free flow of prana, preventing cells from receiving the energy they need. The functioning of chakras is greatly influenced by our thoughts, emotions, perceptions and even intuition. Negative feelings and ideas can create disruptions in the energy flow.

CHAKRA CHARACTERISTICS AND VIBRATIONAL FREQUENCIES

Chakras are associated with specific colours, based on Indian and Eastern philosophies. These colours help individuals understand and work with energy centres. Each chakra's colour corresponds to different vibrational frequencies, making the concept of energy more relatable. However, these vibrations can vary from person to person, depending on their level of awareness. Different traditions may have varying interpretations of chakras and their associated colours, but these vibrational frequencies and colours serve as tools to help individuals become more conscious of their energies and learn to work with them.

Each chakra vibrates at a unique frequency, and it is essential to maintain the chakras at their optimal levels. When the frequency of any particular chakra falls below its required capacity, it disrupts the harmony of all the chakras, leading to erratic behaviour, illnesses and other imbalances. Regular spiritual practice helps keep the chakras aligned and vibrating at the proper frequencies required for a person's overall well-being.

In Vedic science, chakras are often depicted as lotus flowers, each with a different number of petals. The number of petals generally corresponds to the number of nadis that originate from the chakra, giving it the appearance of a lotus. These nadis distribute energy throughout the body. The number of petals also symbolise the vibrational frequency of each chakra. As we ascend from the Mooladhara Chakra to the Sahasrara Chakra, the number of petals increase, signifying a rise in consciousness.

The depiction of chakras as lotus flowers actually symbolises a person's journey from ignorance (darkness) to light, from lower consciousness to higher consciousness. A lotus originates from mud (ignorance), blooms in water and then exists in the air (reaches enlightenment). Similarly, a person's quest for knowledge takes them on a journey from ignorance to light through their efforts and endeavour.

Each chakra has a beeja mantra. A beeja is a seed and just as a seed has the potential to manifest the whole tree, these sounds, when chanted properly, have immense potential to activate and balance the concerned chakra.

Each of the seven major chakras is associated with specific organs and functions within the body. The lower chakras, known as bhoga chakras (energy consumers), are primarily concerned with the emotions and needs of the physical body, making them denser and causing them to vibrate at lower frequencies. In contrast, the upper chakras, known as yoga chakras (energy receivers), are connected to higher spiritual energies, and their activation leads to elevated states of consciousness.

The flow of energy through the chakras determines our overall health and balance. The practice of yoga and meditation aims to balance these energies, purify the lower chakras and guide the energy up towards the higher chakras—this is the requirement for true spiritual awakening. While there are many methods to energise or balance the chakras, true awakening can only occur when karmic imprints are completely eradicated. Karmic imprints refer to the impressions that the atma carries forward from previous births, which need to be exhausted.

The topic of chakras is extensive, but we will not delve into too many details here. The focus now is on understanding how imbalances in the chakras can lead to physical, mental and emotional disturbances, and how mudras can help restore that balance.

THE SEVEN MAJOR CHAKRAS

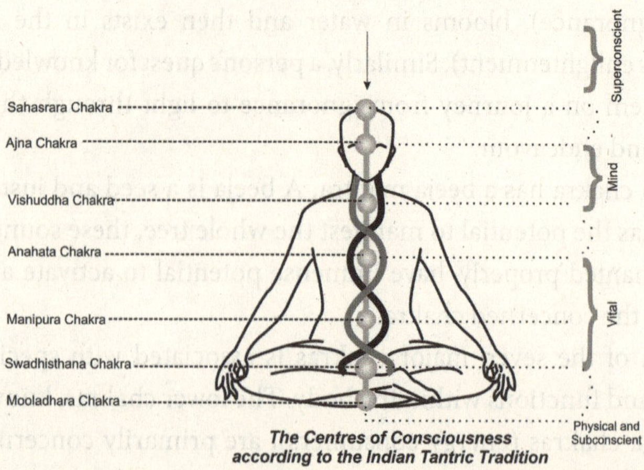

The Centres of Consciousness according to the Indian Tantric Tradition

MOOLADHARA CHAKRA: THE ROOT OF OUR BEING

The Mooladhara Chakra, also known as Root chakra, is located at the base of the spine; specifically, at the tailbone. Moola means root, and adhara means base or support. Mooladhara translates to root support. This chakra lies just below the genital area and above the anus, precisely at the endpoint of the tailbone. It is associated with the colour red and is the seat of Kundalini Shakti, the dormant creative energy within every person.

Kundalini, often depicted as a serpent in a state of deep sleep, is the source of all human energy. The beeja mantra for this chakra, represented within a square mandala, is LAM. Four types of subtle energies are active in this chakra, represented by a lotus with four petals. The Brahma Granthi, or knot of Brahma, is also located here and must be opened through sadhana (spiritual practice) and purification. Energising the Mooladhara Chakra fosters inner stability and balance.

The Mooladhara Chakra is associated with the Prithvi Tatva, and therefore holding the Prithvi Mudra is the ideal gesture to energise it. You may have observed that some individuals, despite having all they need, constantly crave for more. This mindset reflects a sense of scarcity and could indicate a blocked Mooladhara Chakra. Conversely, there are those who embody a sense of abundance even when they have very little.

An imbalanced Mooladhara Chakra may result in:

- Problems in the legs, feet, rectum, tailbone and immune system.
- Issues with the male reproductive system and prostate glands.
- Degenerative arthritis, knee pain, sciatica, eating disorders and constipation.

- Irregular menstrual cycles.
- Stress related to financial security.
- A sense of scarcity, stress and indecisiveness.

Mooladhara Mudra enhances the power of elimination—not just at the physical level, but also at the mental and emotional levels. A woman reported changes in her thought process, and found it easier to let go of the unnecessary people and situations in her life—something she had been struggling with. Since all the fingers are linked, this mudra helps to tap into the energy of all the elements.

For beginners, it is advised to start with Prithvi Mudra to balance the tatva in the chakra. With practice, one can hold the Mooladhara Mudra as shown below:

Hand Formation: Mooladhara Mudra

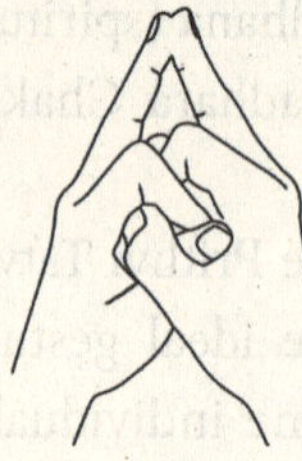

- Bend the ring and little fingers on both hands inward and interlock them.
- The middle fingers of both hands stretch upward and touch each other.
- The index fingers and thumbs of both hands are interlocked.

Benefits:

- As this mudra stimulates the Mooladhara Chakra, it may provide relief from physical pains, aches and cramps in the feet and legs.
- It is good for female reproductive organs. Users of the mudra have claimed to be able to regulate their menstrual cycles and better deal with menopausal issues.
- As it strengthens the base of the spine, it is beneficial for pregnant and postpartum women.

- Practitioners of the mudra have testified that they found relief from pain centred on the lower back and tailbone.
- There have been cases where the mudra has been used to support patients with osteoporosis.
- At the spiritual level, this mudra helps channel energy and thoughts in a positive direction, while also allowing one to tap into their inner potential.
- It helps one develop the ability to let go of undue burdens.
- This chakra is associated with smell, and hence an energised chakra would mean a heightened sense of smell which may result in the practitioner being aware of aromas not easily perceptible to others.

SWADHISTHANA CHAKRA: THE SEAT OF CREATIVITY AND PLEASURE

The Swadhisthana Chakra is located just two fingers above the Mooladhara Chakra, behind the genital organs. The word swa-adhisthana means to abide in one's own abode. It is also known as the Sacral chakra. The chakra is associated with the colour orange and is linked to pleasure experienced through the tongue and genital organs. It is represented by six petals, each corresponding to one of the six subtle energies that operate here. The beeja mantra associated with this chakra is VAM.

At the physical level, this chakra governs the organs of excretion and reproduction, including the lower abdomen and kidneys. Visualising the chakra can aid in addressing disorders related to these organs.

At a deeper level, the Swadhisthana Chakra serves as a repository for all samskaras, or past mental impressions and negativities. These can be cleared through the purification of this chakra. Lower back pain is sometimes a result of the stored emotional and mental baggage associated with this energy centre.

The Swadhisthana Chakra is associated with the Water element. Imbalance in this chakra may manifest as:

- Lack of creativity, initiative and adaptability.
- Over-emotional responses and low self-worth.
- Difficulty staying grounded.
- Varicose veins, kidney and bladder issues, impotence and infertility.

Beginners should focus on Akasha Mudra and then hold the Swadhisthana Mudra.

Hand Formation: Swadhisthana Mudra

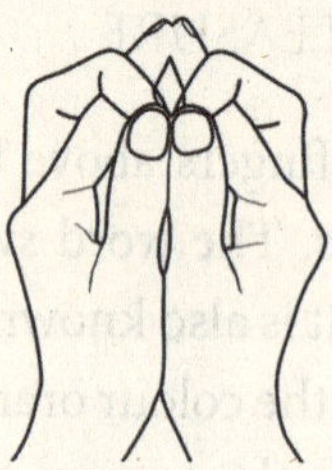

- Hold both palms facing each other, hands touching at the wrists.
- Interlace the little and ring fingers of both hands.
- Bend the middle fingers over the index fingers of the same hand.
- Touch the tips of the middle fingers with the pads of the thumbs on both hands.
- The two index fingers should be touching each other.
- One can start by holding the mudra for three minutes and gradually increase to thirty minutes.

Benefits:

- At the physical level, this mudra could immensely benefit professionals who primarily use their hands and fingers, such as typists, guitarists, drummers, etc.
- It promotes joint flexibility and mobility.

- It is beneficial for the overall reproductive health of both men and women.
- Regular practice of this mudra activates not just the Swadhisthana Chakra but the Ajna and Sahasrara Chakras (Crown chakra) as well, which are associated with spiritual growth and intuition. This helps you connect with the inner self.
- The mudra enhances balance in relationships and encourages one to engage in new experiences.
- It has a calming effect on the body and mind, and one easily enters the 6th and 7th limbs—dharana and dhyanam—of Ashtanga yoga.
- The Swadhisthana Chakra being the seat of creativity, this mudra enables ideas to flow freely, and makes one open to new experiences.

MANIPURA CHAKRA: THE CITY OF JEWELS

The third chakra from the base of the spine is located behind the navel and is known as Manipura, meaning city of jewels. This chakra radiates vitality and energy, symbolised by its fiery yellow colour. It is represented by ten petals, each signifying one of the ten subtle energies at work in this chakra. The beeja mantra associated with Manipura is RAM. This chakra is the centre of self-assertion, dynamism and dominance, embodying ambition, willpower and the ability to lead. It governs the digestive fire and controls the digestive organs, including the pancreas and liver. When the digestive system is out of balance, it can result in sluggishness and depression. Agni Tatva manifests in the body as heat. If the Manipura Chakra functions well, it supplies energy, or heat, to different digestive organs. The Agni Tatva at the Manipura Chakra is called the 'seat of sacred fire' as it governs digestion and metabolism, converting food into energy. To this sacred fire, we offer not just the oblation of food, but also conscious breathing (pranayama). Beyond its physical role, this fire symbolises inner strength, willpower and the capacity for personal transformation, and hence is referred to as sacred fire.

When the energy of this chakra is low, it may manifest as:

- A tendency to view people merely as tools for personal gain.
- Lack of sensitivity and fear of rejection.
- Low self-confidence and self-esteem.
- Digestive disorders.
- Lethargy, inertia and indecisiveness.

Our 'gut feelings' are linked with the Ajna Chakra. A gut feeling is usually an intuition, but it can be led astray by strong emotions and hence become irrational. At the same time, decisions based purely on intellect may not be wise either. Therefore, to arrive at the right decision, we need gut feeling as well viveka (the power of discrimination) to work in tandem, which is attainable through an energised Ajna Chakra. Thus, setting aside the physical benefits, even for spiritual benefits, the gut has to function properly. As the chakra connected to the gut, the Manipura Chakra must be balanced to help us make informed and sound decisions.

Beginners should hold the Surya Mudra and then hold the Manipura Mudra.

Hand Formation: Manipura Mudra

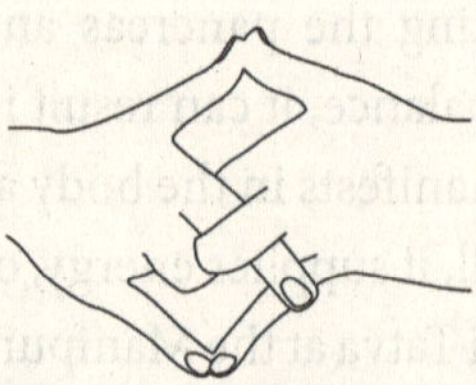

- Hold both hands with palms facing down and fingers stretched out.
- Place the left index finger between the right middle and ring fingers.
- Press the right index finger over the left index finger.

- ☞ Press the left middle finger over the right index finger.
- ☞ Stretch the right index finger to rest over the left little finger.
- ☞ The middle and ring fingers of both hands should be bent down.
- ☞ The little fingers and thumbs of both hands should touch each other.

Benefits:

- ☞ Awakens qualities like self-confidence and awareness, allowing one to live a life free of fear and insecurity.
- ☞ Clarity, wisdom and self-awareness are enhanced once this chakra is energised and blocks are removed. Blocked chakra would mean inability to express thoughts and feelings with coherence, causing one to feel sluggish and drained of energy.
- ☞ Regular practice of this mudra results in better energy levels and enthusiasm. It enhances self-esteem and discipline.
- ☞ In this mudra, all the fingers are interconnected, and hence all the energy circuits are activated.

ANAHATA CHAKRA: THE UNSTRUCK SOUND

This chakra, located at the level of the heart, is known as Anahata, which means unstruck. Anahata-nada, or psychic sound, is the primordial sound, originating from beyond the material world. It resonates in the centre of the heart and is considered the pulse of the universe. The Anahata Chakra is represented by a lotus with twelve petals, symbolising the twelve subtle energies active here. The associated beeja mantra is YAM.

This chakra is green in colour and governs the proper functioning of the heart and the respiratory system. On a deeper level, it is the seat of unconditional love and compassion, representing a state of alertness and awareness. While following the anahata-nada can be joyous, it can also bring sadness. Impurity of mind and thoughts can lead to psychic disorders. If this chakra is imbalanced, stored emotions can rip us apart; impressions of past karmas can surface to disturb the equilibrium of our mind.

An imbalance in this chakra may manifest as:

- Possessiveness, lack of joy, jealousy or even hatred.
- Loneliness and negative thought patterns.
- Health issues such as hypertension, tuberculosis, asthma, palpitations and bronchitis.
- Resistance to new opportunities and frequent feelings of anger.

In the beginning, it is advised to hold the Vayu Mudra, but those with major physical and emotional issues should begin with the Anahata Mudra.

Hand Formation: Anahata Mudra

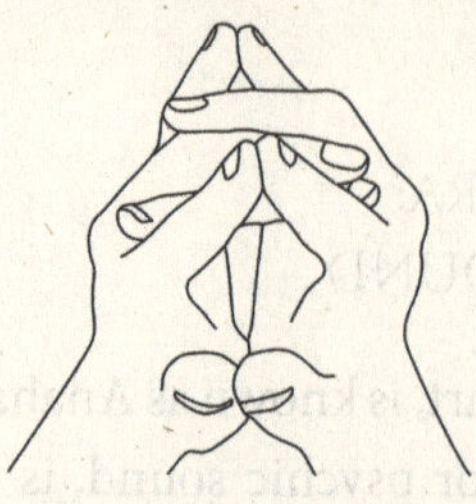

- Touch the little fingers, index fingers and thumbs of both hands with each other.
- The right ring finger is placed on the web between the left index and middle fingers.
- The left ring finger is placed on the web between the right index and middle fingers.
- Curl the two middle fingers.
- This mudra can be held for three to five minutes initially and then gradually increased.
- In this mudra, the Fire, Water and Air elements come into balance, thereby supporting the Anahata Chakra.

Benefits:

- Unwanted emotional bondings and false sense of attachments can be big hurdles on the spiritual path. Feelings of resentment, revenge and possession can bind us. These invariably result in sadness, disorders and a feeling of rejection. This mudra helps free us from emotional bondage.
- An energised chakra would manifest in us in the form of love and compassion for all. The urge to possess or control someone would not arise; one would be able to differentiate between love and possessiveness.
- Emotional cleansing takes place—one would not suffer emotionally from every small incident that occurs.
- At the physical level, the mudra is beneficial for respiratory and cardiovascular health.
- At the spiritual level, this mudra helps purify our mind, helping us connect to the inner self faster.

VISHUDDHA CHAKRA: ABSOLUTE PURITY

This chakra is located at the back of the neck, just behind the throat pit. Blue in colour, it symbolises the acceptance of life's dualities, allowing one to go with the flow and embrace whatever comes. The Sanskrit term vishuddha means absolute purity.

Vishuddha, the seat of communication, balances the physical and subtle energies at the throat centre. It is also the seat for physical and spiritual purification. On a physical level, Vishuddha governs the vocal cords, larynx, and thyroid and parathyroid glands. It is represented by a lotus with sixteen petals, corresponding to the sixteen subtle energies that operate here. The associated beeja mantra is HAM.

An imbalance in this chakra may manifest as:

- Ineffective communication and difficulty expressing oneself.
- Tendency to engage in lies, gossip or to develop addictions.
- Speech and eating disorders.
- Stress, sadness and inner turmoil.
- Reluctance to accept due responsibility for mistakes.

Initially, practitioners should hold Akasha Mudra before holding this mudra.

Hand Formation: Vishuddha Mudra

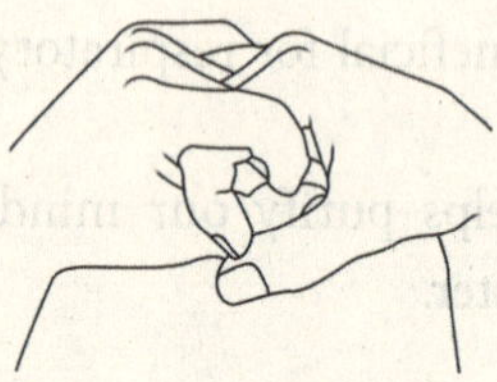

- Hold both palms facing downward, with all the fingers loosely interlocked.
- The index fingers of both hands should be interlocked with the thumb of each respective hand, forming two interlocked circles.
- This mudra should be held for five to forty-five minutes for effective results.

Benefits:

- The element here is Akasha, or Ether—which opens up opportunity for expansion.
- Once the blocks are cleared, an individual feels secure, and is able to trust the people around them.
- Communication is effective and it becomes easier to express emotions. One would no longer run away from problems or deceive oneself.
- The practitioner gets the confidence to overcome obstacles.

- One also develops the confidence necessary to instruct and direct others.

AJNA CHAKRA: THE THIRD EYE

Also known as the third eye, this chakra is located behind the centre of the eyebrows, at the top of the Sushumna Nadi, three to four inches behind the skin surface. If you imagine a line running from the front to the back of the head, intersecting with a line drawn across the top of the ears, the junction inside the brain marks the location of the Ajna Chakra. This is also where the Ida and Pingala Nadis terminate, while the Sushumna Nadi continues upward to the Sahasrara Chakra.

The word ajna means command. It is through this chakra that a seeker receives commands or guidance. As the centre for wisdom and intuition, a purified and awakened Ajna Chakra steadies and strengthens the mind, allowing one to gain full control over prana. It serves as a bridge between the mental and physical realms and is associated with clairvoyance, clairaudience and telepathy. When activated, this chakra enhances mental faculties such as intelligence, memory and concentration, making it possible to send and receive thoughts through this centre. The beeja associated with the chakra is OM.

An imbalance in this chakra may manifest as:

- Lack of clarity and vision.
- Lack of discipline and a poor memory.
- Authoritarian behaviour and arrogance.
- Insomnia, headaches and migraines.

Beginners should hold Jnana Mudra and then start with the Kaleshwara Mudra.

Hand Formation: Kaleshwara Mudra

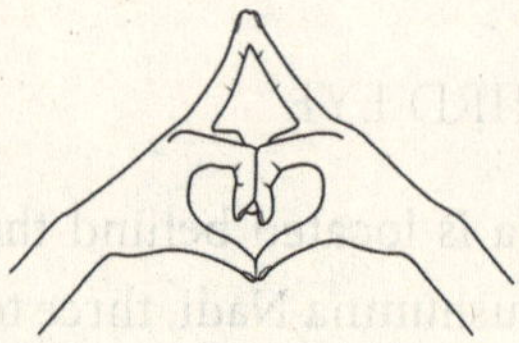

- Hold both palms facing each other.
- Fold all the fingers into the palm.
- The thumbs should touch each other.
- Gently open the middle fingers of both hands so that they touch each other.
- Hold this mudra at the chest level for five to forty-five minutes.

Benefits:

- Energising and unblocking the Ajna Chakra is essential as it helps to understand and connect with the inner self.
- Viveka—power of discrimination—helps one manage emotions, thoughts and feelings that arise from the lower chakras and constantly make one oscillate between thoughts.
- The third eye, when awakened, radiates knowledge that destroys karmic impressions and liberates us from that which is impeding our growth along the spiritual path.
- Once attachments and sorrows are lifted, we feel a sudden shift as clarity of thought prevails. With consistent practice, one may develop the powers of intuition and discernment.

SAHASRARA CHAKRA: THE CROWN CHAKRA

Located at the crown of the head, Sahasrara (thousand-petalled lotus) Chakra is also known as Crown chakra. This is where the fusion of the static (Shiva) and dynamic (Shakti) energy takes place—a process which is known to us as enlightenment, or self-realisation. When the prana shakti reaches this point, it transforms the consciousness completely, leading to experiences that transcend time and space. Individuals have their own karmic journey, but ultimately, one has to reach the same destination. Those who focus on the spiritual path can shorten the journey and one of the ways that can be done is through mudras.

Signs of imbalance in this chakra may include:

- Excessive self-centeredness and lack of inspiration.
- The impression that life is meaningless, which leads to depression.
- Difficulty in connecting with others.

While beginners should focus on Shoonya Mudra, over time, those who wish to focus on spiritual development should hold the Crown, or the Mahamayuri Mudra.

Hand Formation: Crown or Mahamayuri Mudra

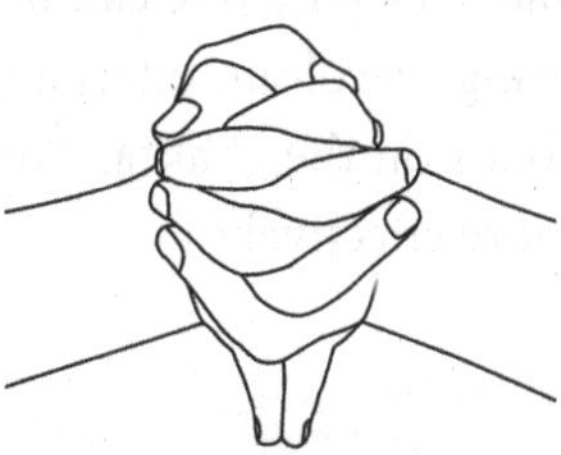

- Join the palms in Pranamam Mudra.
- Press down the right thumb with the left thumb.
- Interlock all fingers except the little fingers.
- Stretch the two little fingers and allow them to touch each other.
- The palms should be softly pressed against each other.
- The hands can be held in front of the stomach or can rest on the lap.

Benefits:

- Activates the Crown chakra, which is associated with spiritual awakening, higher consciousness and transcendence.

- Has a grounding and calming effect, essential for energising the Crown chakra. Along with inner stillness, one experiences relaxation.
- Flow of wisdom is stimulated, thereby also promoting clarity of thought.
- Promotes the functioning of the endocrine glands. Practitioners of the mudra have mentioned relief from hypertension, mood swings, palpitations, sweating, and joint and bone pain.
- Beneficial for the functioning of the pineal gland.
- Users have claimed to experience better sleep patterns and hormonal balance.

***

Each chakra has its own distinct characteristics, including colour, frequency and mantra. To activate a chakra, one can use the corresponding mudra while visualising its colour, internally chanting its mantra and maintaining focus on the chakra. This practice can help alleviate imbalances more effectively.

CHAPTER 5

Pancha Pranas

The Five Vital Forces

In this chapter, we explore how the five vital forces, known as pancha pranas, govern the body and mind. We discover how these energies influence physical, mental and spiritual well-being.

Yoga philosophy states that the human body is capable of experiencing five dimensions of existence, known as the pancha koshas. The physical body that we see is the outermost of the five layers that cover the atman. The five spheres in which a human being lives and experiences are (from gross to subtle): Annamaya Kosha (the food sheath), Pranamaya Kosha (the vital energy sheath), Manomaya Kosha (the mental sheath), Vijnanamaya Kosha (the intellect sheath) and Anandamaya Kosha (the bliss sheath).

According to *Mudra Vigyan*, published by the Bihar School of Yoga, all five sheaths are interconnected with each other; any action or movement in one has a cascading effect on the other sheaths.

Mudras play an important role here as they help create a direct link between three koshas—Pranamaya, Manomaya and Annamaya Koshas. Pranamaya Kosha in particular is responsible for coordinating activities between the Annamaya, Manomaya and Vijnanamaya Koshas. This continuous discharge of pranic force between the koshas, while essential, also creates a dynamic tension. This tension can lead to a person feeling drained mentally and physically, creating imbalance and pranic depletion in every sphere of life. The activation of prana is essential to gain access to the physical, psychic, mental and spiritual dimensions. This is because prana exists in the physical, mental and psychic form and enables us to move from gross to subtle to causal bodies.

However, our ancient sages recognised the need to rebalance the pranic flow. To achieve this, mudras were adopted as an important tool. These mudras help connect the Annamaya Kosha to the other koshas. They have been aptly described as psychological locks (or seals) to redirect the flow of prana. Through regular practice, mudra practitioners can develop an awareness of how prana flows, and can adjust it throughout all the other koshas. Mudras also enable the redirection of prana to the upper chakras and the higher states of consciousness.

UNDERSTANDING PRANA

The term prana does not refer to mechanical breathing. In the words of Swami Chinmayananda (2013), 'it is the manifestation of life in our body' (p. 51). Once prana enters our system, it is divided into different types, each with specific functions. The pancha pranas, or five vital forces, operate like separate departments, each responsible for distinct functions within the body.

These pancha pranas—Prana, Apana, Samana, Udana and Vyana—are the primary forces that continuously operate within the human body. They energise every action, from the movement of the hands to the secretion of digestive juices. These pranas flow through the organs, the mind and the pancha tatvas, playing a crucial role in creation and existence at the individual level. They maintain balance between the physical and mental planes. Understanding the different flows of prana within the system can help us identify issues related to intake, assimilation, digestion, distribution and growth.

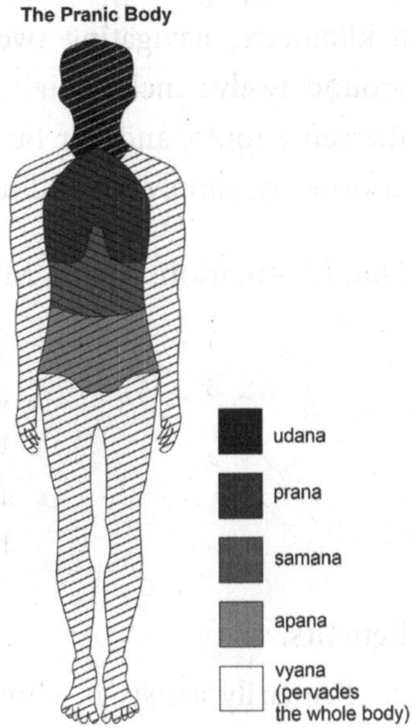

APANA PRANA: THE DOWNWARD FLOW

Apana Prana represents downward-flowing vital energy (vayu) in the pelvic region, extending from the navel to the perineum. It affects the Swadhisthana and Mooladhara Chakras, stimulating the nourishing energy in the pelvic floor.

Function:

Toxins are a major cause of poor health in people. The primary function of Apana Prana is to eliminate toxins and unwanted waste from the body. Apana Prana governs excretion, elimination, reproduction, immunity, bowel movement and the release of bodily fluids such as sweat and urine.

This mudra is highly beneficial for hikers. A woman with known blood pressure issues and a tendency towards asthma went on a pilgrimage that involved walking downhill for about a kilometre, navigating twenty to twenty-five old steps, each around twelve inches high. She then had to walk back along the same route, and her husband was amazed to see she did it effortlessly, simply by holding the Apana Mudra!

Hand Formation: Apana Mudra

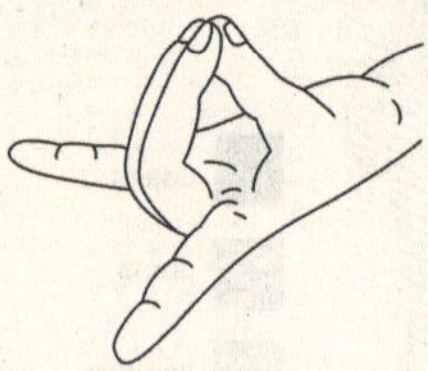

- Touch the tips of the middle finger and ring finger to the tip of the thumb.
- Keep the other two fingers straight but relaxed.

Benefits:

- Primarily assists in eliminating waste and toxins from the body.
- Has a soothing and relaxing effect on the body.
- Users of this mudra have claimed it helps alleviate constipation and gastritis. They have also reported it aids with the expulsion of gases, wind, faeces and urine.
- Since this is a downward-flowing prana, it helps prevent vayu from moving upward towards the abdomen. Hence, it might reduce hiccups, belching and similar conditions.
- Those who use the mudra have observed that it is effective for UTIs and other urinary issues.
- Based on claims by mudra practitioners, it is beneficial for those who have recently been diagnosed with diabetes. According to them, the Apana Mudra should be practised for fifteen minutes, followed by Prana Mudra for another fifteen. Lifelong practice may be necessary for maintenance. It may not be as effective for long-term diabetics.

- Helps expel negative thoughts, and has a balancing effect on the mind, which is closely related to a well-functioning liver.
- At the mental level, it enhances the ability to develop clear vision, leading to serenity and harmony.
- Apana Mudra supports many functions related to the kidneys, bladder, bowels and excretory organs.
- When synchronised with breathing, this mudra can have a calming and relaxing effect.
- Feedback from a few mudra practitioners say it is effective in overcoming addictions such as smoking and drinking, as it alters taste perceptions and reduces cravings.
- Users have conveyed that it has proven beneficial for hikers or anyone experiencing breathlessness, especially if held for ten minutes before climbing.
- Observations from mudra practitioners suggest that it is beneficial for reproductive health. It is recommended that pregnant women practise the mudra for five to ten minutes daily, starting just a month before the due date.
- This is the only mudra recommended for practice immediately after eating, for ten minutes, as it reportedly aids in the expulsion of metabolic by-products.

Contraindications:

- The straight little finger may cause excessive urination.
- Those suffering from colitis or loose motion should avoid this mudra.
- The mudra increases vata and kapha dosha while reducing pitta dosha. Therefore, those with the former two should engage in this mudra in moderation.
- Pregnant women should avoid this mudra for the first eight months as this encourages a downward-flowing prana.

PRANA PRANA: THE INWARD FLOW

Prana shakti, or the life-force energy, regulates the activities of various sense organs. To avoid confusion with the all-pervasive prana, this specific form of prana is also known as Sthoola Prana. Prana Prana refers to the energy currents located in the thoracic region between the diaphragm and the base of the neck. As we breathe, we draw in the life-force energy, which always flows inward and resides in the nasal passage, heart and lungs.

Function:

Prana Prana governs eating, breathing, drinking and mental experiences.

Hand Formation: Prana Mudra

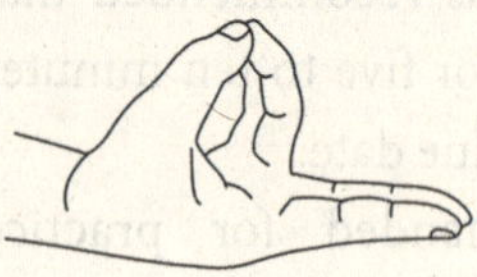

☞ Lightly touch the tips of little finger and ring finger with the tip of thumb.

☞ Keep all the other fingers straight but relaxed.

☞ Rest your hands with the palms facing upward on the knees.

Benefits:

☞ Combines Prithvi and Jala Tatvas, enhancing strength, immunity, vitality and stamina.

☞ There are claims that it helps address vitamin deficiencies, overcome weakness, increase circulation and reduce bad odour.

☞ Many use the mudra to control hunger and thirst, especially when fasting.

☞ Beneficial for the lungs and eyes. User feedback suggests that it is good for thyroid disorders, food allergies and measles.

☞ Supports respiration and swallowing.

- Reported to help reduce muscle cramps and stiffness.
- Promotes strength, courage, focus and intuitive knowledge.
- Especially beneficial for those with kapha constitution, as it balances the Water and Earth elements of kapha.
- Reduces mental tension, forgetfulness, irritability and jealousy by alleviating negative emotions.
- For removal of air trapped in the joints, hold the Vayu Mudra for thirty minutes, followed by the Prana Mudra for another thirty.
- Clears the pathways of prana, improving lung function and oxygen intake, enhancing concentration and clearing thought processes.
- This mudra, when practised in conjunction with other therapeutic mudras, can amplify their positive effects.
- Considered safe, with no specific precautions necessary.
- For best results, this mudra should be practised at the end of the day for ten minutes, unless it is a part of a prescribed mudra therapy regimen.

Contraindication:

- Should be avoided by individuals with excessive kapha dosha, as it may further increase kapha while reducing pitta dosha.

UDANA PRANA: THE SPIRALLING FLOW

Udana Prana operates from the neck to the top of the head, and extends to the arms and legs. It can be felt as spiralling flows of energy that empower the body in various ways.

Function:

This vital energy provides the neck with the strength necessary to support the head, and enables the vocal cords to vibrate, facilitating speech. Udana Prana also coordinates and controls the movements of the legs, arms and neck, playing a crucial role in physical balance and coordination. It pervades the Ajna, Bindu and Sahasrara Chakras, influencing higher consciousness and mental clarity.

Hand Formation: Udana Mudra

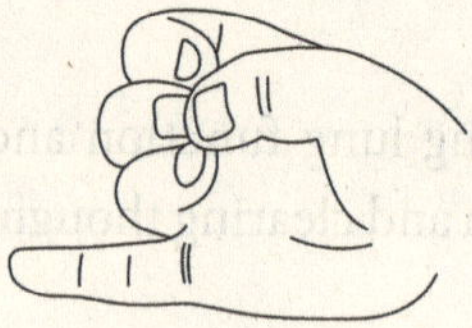

- Bring the tips of the thumb, index, middle and ring fingers together.
- Keep the little finger straight.
- Rest the hands on the knees, palms facing upward.

Benefits:

- Supports the health of tonsils, throat and vocal cords, and is sometimes beneficial for addressing speech-related problems, though it cannot rectify congenital issues.
- Enhances brain function by flooding it with fresh oxygen, keeping the mind alert and active.
- Activates the Vishuddha Chakra, which is associated with communication and self-expression.
- It has been reported to provide relief from headaches.
- Promotes kidney health.
- Governs thoughts and consciousness.
- Udana Mudra harmonises and activates limbs and the associated nerves, ligaments, joints and muscles, helping to maintain an erect posture.
- Induces a sense of joy and lightness in the body.
- Mudra users have claimed that it is beneficial for the health of the thyroid and parathyroid glands.
- Helps in clearing misconceptions and wrong notions.

This mudra not only aids in physical health, but also contributes to mental clarity and spiritual well-being, making it a valuable practice for overall balance and harmony.

VYANA PRANA: THE CIRCULATING PRANA

Vyana Prana circulates across the body, distributing energy from the digested food to areas where it is needed most. For example, an athlete requires more energy, specifically in the legs, while running.

Function:

Vyana Prana acts as a reserve force for other pranas.

Hand Formation: Vyana Mudra

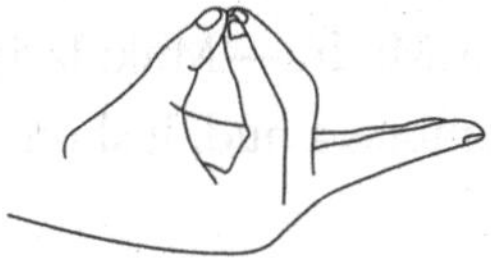

- Touch the tips of the index and middle fingers to the tip of the thumb.
- Keep the other fingers straight.
- Rest the hands on the knees with the palms facing upward.

Benefits:

- Facilitates the circulation of blood throughout the body, determining the force with which it flows through veins and arteries.
- Supports the movement of various enzymes and hormones.
- Practitioners often report that the mudra regulates blood pressure, oxygenates cells and is a remedy for body stiffness.
- Enhances the function of different organs.
- Coordinates and controls movements, harmonising the actions of other prana vayus.

- Governs the circulation of nutrients and muscular movements.
- Users have reported that the mudra aids in managing sunstroke, excessive sleep and saliva secretion, and helps maintain appropriate body temperature.
- It is credited with helping to overcome lethargy and providing mental stability.
- Promotes a healthy digestive system by supporting jatharagni, the digestive fire.

SAMANA PRANA: THE SIDEWAYS FLOWING PRANA

A healthy life begins with a healthy stomach. Samana Prana is a balancing energy that flows sideways—from the navel to the diaphragm. The term samana means equal or balanced, indicating its role as an equaliser or balancer; it balances all the five elements. It is also known as Mukula Mudra—Mukula in Sanskrit meaning bud—as this mudra resembles a bud. It should be held for at least fifteen minutes.

Function:

Samana Prana is one of the pancha vayus responsible for aiding digestion. It manages the digestive system and prepares food for absorption by the body. When Samana Prana is balanced, it helps the body absorb and retain what is beneficial while eliminating what is unnecessary. It ensures that the digestive fire remains active and does not diminish. Samana Prana governs digestion, secretion and metabolism.

I have feedback from several patients on the use of Samana Mudra for different purposes. For instance, a woman suffering from glaucoma found that holding the Samana Mudra over the eyes for fifteen minutes daily helped bring down her eye pressure to a normal range. Another patient with retinal degeneration reported immense relief from the very first instance they began holding this mudra over the eyes. Calluses on the feet due to bunions can be very painful. A patient mentioned that at times, she would get shooting pains in that area. She tried my suggestion of rubbing the area in Samana Mudra and found quick relief.

Hand Formation: Samana (Mukula) Mudra

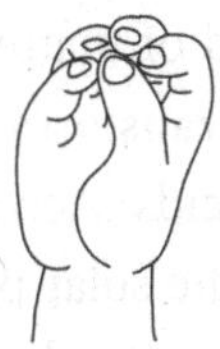

- Bring the tips of all the fingers together to resemble a bud.
- Place your palms facing upward, with hands resting on the knees.

Benefits:

- Users of the mudra have reported that it helps with acidity and aids in the absorption of nutrients.
- Strengthens the functioning of the liver, stomach, duodenum, spleen, and both the small and large intestines.
- Practitioners often state that it is beneficial for skin disorders, including acne, blackheads, pimples and leukoderma.
- Balances all the elements in the body.
- When Samana Prana is balanced, the mudra helps absorb and retain what is needed while eliminating unnecessary elements.
- Keeps the jatharagni active.
- Contributes to a healthy digestive system—it is recommended that we eat with all five fingers to balance all the tatvas.
- Enhances experiences of the mind.
- Several mudra users consider it a simple but effective way of pain relief. Hold the mudra over the area which is injured or in pain. For shoulder pain, rub the hand in a clockwise

motion over your shoulders while holding the Samana Mudra, and place the other hand on a knee (holding the mudra). This helps concentrate the generated energy at one point, providing instant relief.

☞ It provides vitality and dynamism.

THE ROLE OF FIRE (AGNI) IN HEALTH

Fire is an active energy that transforms one kind of matter into another. Jatharagni, the digestive fire within us, transforms food into essential nutrients like oxygen and amino acids. According to the *Shiva Samhita* (2.33), this fire, located at the solar plexus, performs various metabolic functions. It is described as the destroyer of disease and the bestower of longevity, vitality, nourishment and swiftness in the body.

Therefore, an intelligent yogi should ignite the Vaisvanara fire daily and offer food as an oblation under the guidance of a preceptor (*Shiva Samhita*, 2.34).

Pranas and Digestion

Imbalances in any of the pranas can affect digestion. Free flow of pranas nourishes your whole body—muscles, nerves, cells and organs—enhancing vitality and dynamism.

Two shlokas from the Bhagavad Gita are traditionally chanted before meals to honour the role of pranas in digestion. The first is:

ब्रह्मार्पणं ब्रह्म हविर्ब्रह्माग्नौ ब्रह्मणा हुतम् ।
ब्रह्मैव तेन गन्तव्यं ब्रह्मकर्मसमाधिना ॥ ४-२४॥

brahmārpaṇaṃ brahma havirbrahmāgnau brahmaṇā hutam |
brahmaiva tena gantavyaṃ brahmakarmasamādhinā || 4.24 ||

The act of offering, the offering itself and the sacred fire are all manifestations of Brahman. True liberation is attained by one who realises this truth—that Brahman is what is to be perceived and attained. He alone sees Brahman in all things.

The relationship of pranas and digestion has been beautifully explained in shloka 14 of chapter 15 in the Bhagavad Gita:

अहं वैश्वानरो भूत्वा प्राणिनां देहमाश्रितः ।
प्राणापान- समायुक्तः पचाम्यन्नं- चतुर्विधम्- ॥ 15.14 ॥

ahaṃ vaiśvānaro bhūtvā prāṇināṃ dehamāśrita- ḥ |
prāṇāpāna- samāyuktaḥ pacāmyannaṃ- caturvidham- || 15.14 ||

I am the fire of digestion in every living body, says Bhagavan. I am the air of life, outgoing (Apana) and incoming (Prana), by which I digest the four kinds of food. Chaturvidham (four ways food is consumed)—chewing, sucking, drinking and licking.

Fire (Agni) and Its Functions

- Manages metabolism, digestion, body temperature, vision and blood temperature.
- Provides heat, light and energy.
- Governs digestion, sense of sight and muscle function.
- On an emotional level, it enhances inner strength, willpower, self-esteem, self-confidence, courage, ambition and integrity.

Connection Between Mantras, Mudras and Digestion

Certain mantras and mudras are used in temples while offering naivedyam (food offering). While the sages ritualised these practices, the purpose is to invoke the pancha pranas for better digestion and assimilation. When pancha pranas are invoked through mantras while holding the related mudra, they activate the koshas and energies. As a child, I watched my grandfather perform a ritual before he began his meals. Once the thali was served and placed before him, he would mentally offer an oblation of each item, placing it on the top right corner of the thali. He would then take a few drops of water in his right palm, and encircle the thali in a clockwise direction, lightly sprinkling the water around it before pouring it over the offered food. Today, I understand this as parishinchami, a purification ritual performed before eating.

Prana is the life-force energy and koshas are different dimensions of consciousness. The Pranamaya Kosha organises body parts; it is responsible for regulating the prana and ensuring that all the systems in our body function harmoniously. It provides movement for physical and mental expression. The Pranamaya Kosha consists of five major pranas, each linked to a specific system in the body. As we chant, we evoke these respective systems:

Om Pranaya Swaha (The respiratory system)

Om Apanaya Swaha (The excretory system)

Om Vyanaya Swaha (The circulatory system)

Om Udanaya Swaha (The sensory system)

Om Samanaya Swaha (The digestive system)

It is recommended that one consumes the first five morsels of food while chanting each of these mantras. Acharya Keshav Dev suggests using the ring finger, little finger and thumb (as in Prana Mudra) while consuming food, if one has vitamin deficiency or to regain lost energy.

CHAPTER 6

Vibhaga Pranayama Mudras

Yoga Shastra, *Garuda Purana* and *Dhyana Bindu Upanishad* all state that a human being takes 21,600 breaths over the course of twenty-four hours. A person should ideally breathe fifteen times per minute. This equates to 900 breaths per hour and 21,600 breaths per day. According to science journalist James Nestor (2020), it takes an average person 3.3 seconds to inhale and exhale (p. 28). Siddha science tells us that by reducing the number of breaths—or alternatively, by increasing the duration of a single breath—we can reduce our breathing rate, which in turns supports a longer lifespan, although this can vary among individuals. In fact, slow breathing is associated with a calm and serene mind.

BREATHING AND LUNG CAPACITY

Total Lung Capacity (TLC) is the volume of air in the lungs after maximum inspiration effort. Among healthy adults, the average lung capacity is 5.8 litres. However, most people typically use just about one-third of it.

Almost everyone breathes without thinking, and many do so incorrectly, using only a small portion of their respiratory capacity. Modern lifestyle changes have impacted proper breathing practices. Shallow breathing deprives the body of oxygen and prana, while irregular breathing disrupts the normal flow of prana, causing mental and emotional blocks.

Emotions, thoughts and imagination affect breathing, as do dietary changes and stress, which can deplete energy levels; when the mind is agitated, breathing becomes rapid. Both pain and exercise also influence the breathing process.

Making a habit of breathing correctly is essential not only for vitality but also for disease prevention. Rhythmic, slow and deep respiration leads to a calm and contented state of mind. Proper breathing enhances resistance to diseases—it is said that our time on earth depends on the number of breaths we take per minute. According to the yogacharya B.K.S. Iyengar (2016), 'The yogi's life is not measured in the number of his days but in the number of his breaths' (p. 43). In addition to physical health, proper breathing ensures happiness, self-control, clear-sightedness and spiritual growth.

PRANA AND PRANAYAMA

Breathing is more than just the intake of air. According to James Nestor (2020), 'The tens of billions of molecules we bring into our bodies with every breath ... influence nearly every internal organ ... affect heart rate, digestion, moods, attitudes; when we feel aroused, and when we feel nauseated' (p. 128). The air we breathe is charged with prana, which we extract and use for various purposes. When we breathe normally, we draw in an average amount of prana from the air. But through pranayama, we become capable of extracting a greater supply. This is then stored in the brain and nerve centres for later use. The action not only strengthens different parts of the body but also increases brain energy. A person who practises pranayama radiates vitality and strength, and can even transfer this energy to others.

Thus, pranayama may be understood, in essence, as the control of prana by regulating our breathing habits using certain techniques and practices. Regulated, rhythmic respiration purifies the body and quietens the mind. While breathing is usually an unconscious (involuntary) process, we can take control of it and make it a conscious (voluntary) activity.

VIBHAGA PRANAYAMA MUDRAS

Various methods have been suggested by different schools of thought to regulate breathing—and thus, prana—and mudra vijnana has its own specific methods. The word vibhaga means sectional. When one practises Vibhaga Pranayama Mudras, one experiences the union (yoga) of breath and mind. Thus, pranayama is a state of yoga that is attained through regulated breathing.

The lungs have three sections—the right lung has three lobes, while the left lung has two; the heart is located at the mid-lobe region. The sections of the lungs are:

- Adhama: the lower, or inferior, abdominal area.
- Madhyama: the intercostal (ribcage) region, or the middle portion.
- Adyama: the clavicular (collar bone) region, or the superior area.

Accordingly, there are three types of breathing methods—diaphragmatic, thoracic and clavicular breathing techniques. Vibhaga pranayama helps in sectional breathing control. Our normal breathing is very shallow and happens at the upper chest level, and hence only the upper lobes of the lungs are filled. Sectional breathing can help correct this breathing pattern and increase lung capacity by encouraging proper airflow into different areas of the lungs. It teaches us how to hold and regulate the breath within each of the three sections.

Vibhaga pranayama improves the health of the lungs and helps oxygenate more and more cells in the body by facilitating the absorption of an abundant supply of oxygen. In sectional breathing, our focus is on different parts of the lungs, and hence our overall awareness of breathing pattern is enhanced. This also means more toxins are released. In shallow breathing, carbon dioxide and other toxins are not completely released from the system. Conscious, deep breathing stimulates the lymphatic system, which helps release toxins from the body. Deep breathing results in better blood flow, which in turn helps transport waste matter smoothly to the organs responsible for elimination or detoxification. These benefits can be achieved through four mudras coupled with conscious deep breathing.

Yogis like B.K.S. Iyengar classify respiration into four types. Corresponding to these different types, there are four different Vibhaga Pranayama Mudras for different methods of respiration:

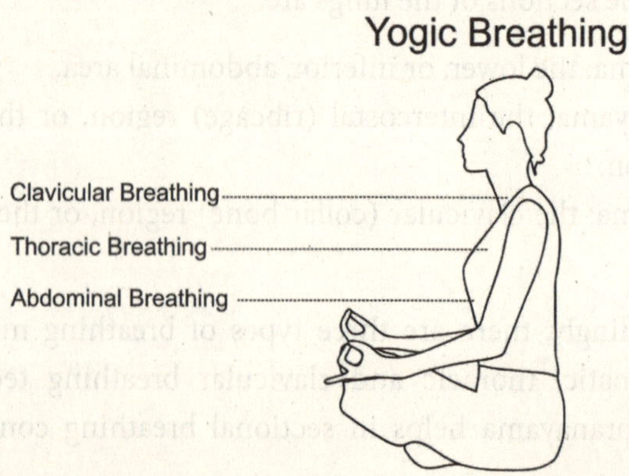

1. Low breathing (Adhama): Chin Mudra for diaphragmatic breathing.
2. Mid breathing (Madhyama): Chinmaya Mudra for thoracic breathing.
3. High breathing (Adya): Adi Mudra for clavicular breathing
4. Yogi complete breathing: Brahma Mudra for Poorna pranayama.

CHIN MUDRA: DIAPHRAGMATIC BREATHING (ADHAMA)

This is the most natural and efficient way of breathing. It fills the lower part of the lungs. The diaphragm rises upward in the chest cavity during exhalation. During inhalation, it moves downward, creating more space in the chest cavity. Thus, as the diaphragm is used during respiration, it enhances the lung capacity. Apart from filling up the lower part of the lungs, diaphragmatic breathing also stimulates the liver, stomach, intestines and other organs that lie just beneath it. In addition, it has a positive effect on cardiac function.

Initially, for the first two to three breaths, you may need to make a conscious effort to achieve this, but soon it will become automatic. Respiration should be smooth.

Hand Formation:

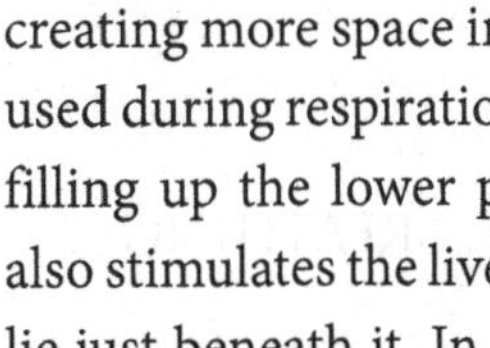

☞ On both hands, lightly touch the tip of the thumb to that of the index finger.

☞ Keep the other fingers straight but relaxed.

☞ Place your hands on your thighs, palms facing down.

☞ Hold this mudra for five minutes.

Benefits:

- Mudra practitioners claim it is beneficial for regulating blood pressure.
- Strengthens the nervous system.
- Enhances blood circulation.
- Reduces water content in the legs and feet.
- Promotes the health of the eyes.
- Supports better sleeping patterns.
- Can be of use when healing strain in the vocal box.
- Activates Apana Vayu; you might feel the abdomen expanding and contracting.
- Promotes positive thoughts.
- Increases memory power as energy flows back to the brain through the nerves.
- Reduces mental tension.

CHINMAYA MUDRA: THORACIC BREATHING (MADHYAMA)

In the thoracic breathing method, the breath is directed to the middle region of the lungs. The ribcage expands and contracts. Chinmaya Mudra influences prana and affects respiration by stimulating movement in the thoracic region. Energy is directed into the areas of Samana and Prana, between the navel and the throat, leading to a new state of harmony.

Hand Formation:

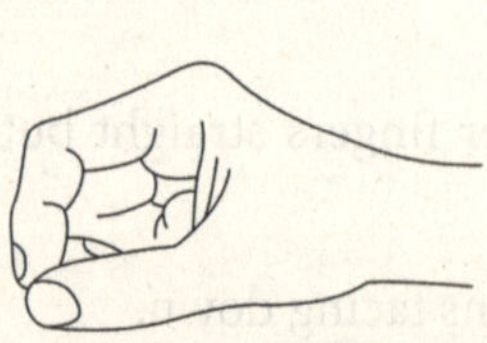

- On both hands, touch the tips of the thumb and index fingers together.
- Place your hand on your thighs with your palms facing down.

- Curl the other three fingers into the palm.
- Hold this for five minutes.

Benefits:

- Users of this mudra have reported that it is good for the heart, alleviates joint pains, slows the breathing rate and reduces stress.
- Increases awareness, helping one identify the source of stress and anxiety.
- Improves the nervous system and regulates the digestive system. It is also reported to help relieve constipation.
- Aids in relieving stress, which in turn helps alleviate arthritis.
- Reported to stimulate the release of serotonin, a mood stabiliser, leading to relaxation and pain relief.

ADI MUDRA: CLAVICULAR BREATHING (ADYA)

The word adi means beginning, and this is the first mudra that a foetus forms. Clavicular breathing involves shallow breathing, and air is drawn into the upper region of the lungs. The ribs are elevated, and the collarbone and shoulders rise up. The upper ribs and collarbones are pulled upward by the muscles of the neck, throat and sternum. This type of breathing typically occurs under conditions of extreme physical exertion or when experiencing obstructive respiratory diseases such as asthma. Adi Mudra balances Udana Vayu, stimulating both Prana and Udana. Udana stimulates the functioning and development of the sense organs and has a calming effect on the nervous system. It increases the capacity of the upper lobes of the lungs. The mudra requires all the fingers to be closed, and hence the loss of prana is minimised.

Hand Formation:

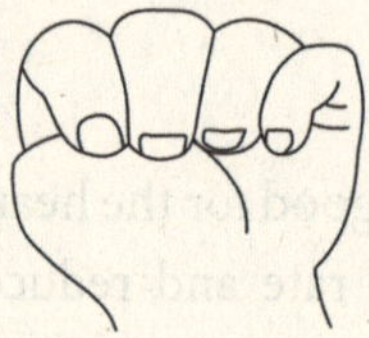

- Place the tip of thumb at the base of the little finger.
- Close all the other fingers over the thumb.
- Place your hands on your thighs with the palms down.

Benefits:

- The mudra can support sports enthusiasts, especially those with cervical spondylitis.
- Supplies energy to the jnanendriyas, enhancing the corresponding elements and making communication—speech, hearing, etc.—easier.
- Reduces anxiety and tension while boosting confidence.
- Activates the neurons in the brain.
- Activates the Anahata and Vishuddha Chakras.
- Reported to reduce snoring.
- Increases oxygen flow and improves lung capacity.
- Enhances your ability to connect with the inner self.
- Calms the nervous system.
- Stimulates the intellect and increases attention span.
- Enhances concentration and heightens awareness.

Contraindication:

- Those with high blood pressure issues should not practise this for more than five minutes.

BRAHMA MUDRA: POORNA PRANAYAMA

This mudra combines all three types of sectional breathing. It involves holding the mudra and inhaling sequentially—starting with inhalation from the diaphragm, followed by the thoracic and clavicular regions. Exhale in the reverse sequence. Repeat this process five times.

Hand Formation:

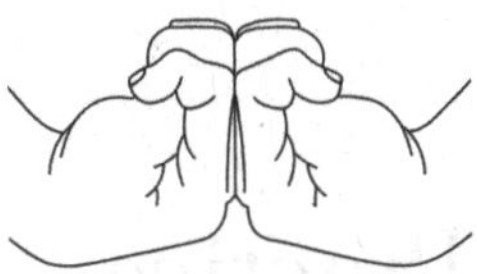

- Begin by holding the Adi Mudra.
- Bring the knuckles of both hands together.
- Press the hands against the pubic bone, palms facing up.

Benefits:

- The lungs are completely filled.
- Enhances your ability to connect with the inner self.
- Improves the movement of the diaphragm, chest and collarbones.
- Brings harmony to all five elements within the body.
- The positioning of both hands together brings balance to the left and right sides of the body.
- Placement of the hands at the pubic bone redirects the flow of prana upward along the spine, from the lower chakras to the higher chakras.

All the Vibhaga Pranayama Mudras should be practised while sitting in a relaxed and comfortable manner. Breathe only through the nose.

CHAPTER 7

Mudras for Daily Practice

The human body is complete in itself. However, to remain in good health, it is necessary to maintain a balance of the pancha tatvas, and practising mudras is one of the easiest and safest ways to do this. Those with no ailments can perform certain mudras daily to sustain their well-being. If done regularly, these mudras, prescribed by ancient texts, help maintain both physical and mental health. From my years of experience, I have found that practising mudras with dedication and faith can truly support overall health and well-being. The prescribed mudras should be practised for ten minutes daily, either in one sitting or spaced out throughout the day.

JNANA MUDRA

Referred to as the mudra of wisdom, this mudra balances the Vayu Tatva within the body. This is one of the most widely practised and recognised mudras due to its simplicity and effectiveness.

It is commonly used in meditation; it helps calm the mind and enhances mental clarity.

Jnana Mudra is deeply symbolic. The three open fingers represent the trigunas—the three attributes of prakriti, namely sattwa, rajas and tamas. These are the three fundamental attributes of creation. Sattwa represents understanding, purity and light; rajas symbolises action, passion and dynamism; tamas signifies inertia, darkness and ignorance. Through regular practice of the Jnana Mudra, one can transcend all the three states progressively, and travel from darkness and ignorance to light and higher knowledge.

When holding the Jnana Mudra, the thumb represents universal consciousness (Brahman), while the index finger symbolises individual consciousness (Atman). The contact between these fingers signifies the union of the individual and the universe, harmonising and balancing the body's energy levels. The other three fingers remain extended but separate, conveying the detachment of the individual consciousness from the three attributes of nature (Prakriti).

The pineal and pituitary glands, two small but crucial glands located within the brain, play vital roles in the overall health of the body, and particularly that of the endocrine system. The thumb contains the pressure points capable of affecting both these glands, and their stimulation in Jnana Mudra has far-reaching effects.

The concept of pineal gland, often referred to as the 'third eye', is rooted in various spiritual texts. It is associated with the Ajna Chakra, which is considered the centre of intuition, higher consciousness and insight. The pineal gland helps enhance the production of melatonin, thereby improving sleep quality and regulating sleep-wake cycles. This, in turn, promotes relaxation and reduces stress.

Stimulation of the pituitary gland is crucial for regulating various hormonal functions in the body. This can lead to the improvement of our overall health and well-being, particularly due to the resultant balancing effect on our growth, metabolism, reproductive processes and stress response.

Hand Formation:

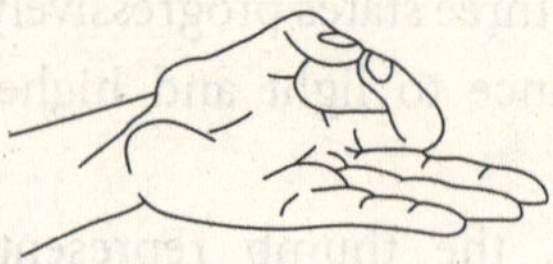

- Lightly touch the tips of the index finger and thumb, forming a circle.
- Keep the other three fingers close together and extended, but relaxed.
- Place the hands on your knees. This completes a circuit of energy, enhancing the flow of prana throughout the body.

Benefits:

- The connection between the index finger and thumb creates an energy circuit that directs the prana back through the body and up to the brain, fostering focus and mental clarity.
- Placing the hands on the knees stimulates a Gupt nadi that runs from the knees, through the inside of the thighs, and up to the perineum. This energy, which would have otherwise dissipated, now travels through the body and activates the Mooladhara Chakra.
- The upward-facing palms stimulate the nerves along the inner arms, opening up the lungs and chest cavity, thereby enhancing respiratory function and boosting lung capacity.
- The Jnana Mudra, according to practitioners, can improve mental disorders, and alleviate stress and anxiety. It is also known to sharpen memory and concentration, and hence

is suitable for anyone seeking mental clarity, particularly students and professionals.

- Regular practice of this mudra is suggested to help with insomnia, depression, sleep disorders and blood pressure.
- It fosters inner peace, self-insight and overall spiritual development.

SHOONYA VAYU MUDRA

Shoonya Vayu Mudra is a powerful hand gesture that combines the benefits of two mudras: Shoonya Mudra and Vayu Mudra. This mudra is particularly effective for balancing the Vayu Tatva and the Shoonya Tatva in the body. Its practice is highly effective in addressing a wide range of issues.

Hand Formation:

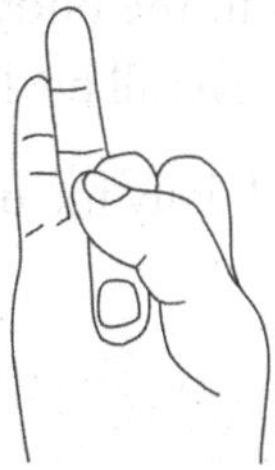

- Fold the index and middle fingers and press the tip of these fingers straight down so that they touch the base of the thumb.
- Gently press on these two fingers with the thumb.
- Keep the other two fingers extended, but relaxed.

Benefits:

- Improves the sleep cycle by calming the mind and balancing the nervous system. It promotes relaxation, making it easier to fall asleep and maintain a restful state.
- Boosts energy levels and enhances stamina, making it an excellent practice for those experiencing fatigue or a general lack of vitality; helps in rejuvenating the body and mind.

- Reduces feelings of indecisiveness and impatience. Helps in fostering a sense of clarity, patience and inner peace, enabling better decision-making.
- Multiple practitioners have claimed that it is beneficial for throat-related problems such as hoarseness, stammering or other voice issues. It helps in soothing the throat, improving vocal clarity and supporting overall throat health.
- The mudra is said to help with pain relief, particularly earache, tooth pain and headache. According to users of the mudra, it works by balancing the Air element in the body, reducing inflammation, thus relieving pain in the affected areas.
- According to various testimonials, it promotes better blood circulation, addressing numbness and tingling sensations in various parts of the body.
- Regular practice of Shoonya Vayu Mudra for at least fifteen minutes daily may help in preventing various illnesses by maintaining the balance of the pancha tatvas in the body. It strengthens the immune system and supports overall health.

The other four mudras that should be practised daily include:

Prithvi Mudra (Refer to Chapter 3)

Akasha Mudra (Refer to Chapter 3)

Apana Mudra (Refer to Chapter 5)

Prana Mudra (Refer to Chapter 5)

CHAPTER 8

Curative Mudras

From my personal experience as well as the feedback I have received from other patients, I can attest that mudras can work. Certain mudras work instantly, some may not, while some may need to be performed for a long duration, especially for chronic cases. Curative mudras need to be done only when necessary and must be discontinued once the problem is resolved.

RESPIRATORY SYSTEM

APANA VAYU (HRIDAYA) MUDRA

Apana Vayu Mudra is a therapeutic mudra and is done with one or both hands. It also operates as a detoxification mudra—with Fire and Ether being the main elements that are affected—and this property has led to it sometimes being known as Mrta Sanjivani Mudra (one that brings the dead back to life). It is also called Hridaya Mudra, as it is beneficial for cardiovascular health. The mudra also supports relief from emotional distress or heartbreak.

There are reports that it can help with certain disorders of the heart. One known incidence is that of a woman who had been admitted to the ICU for heart palpitations and anxiety. She later attended one of my sessions and learnt of this mudra. The next time she faced the exact same situation, she had the presence of mind to open her notes, locate the mudra and hold it. She later testified that within ten minutes she found herself completely alright and free of any distress.

Hand Formation:

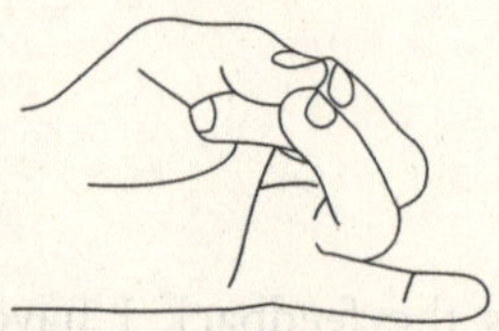

- ☞ As the name suggests, it is a combination of two mudras—the Apana Mudra and the Vayu Mudra.
- ☞ Fold the index finger to touch the base of the thumb (Vayu Mudra).
- ☞ Press down upon the folded index finger with the thumb.
- ☞ Touch the tips of the middle finger and the ring finger to the tip of thumb.

Benefits:

- ☞ Promotes cardiovascular health and diverts the flow of prana from the hands to the heart.
- ☞ Relieves emotional heartache, anxiety, panic, grief, sadness and feelings of being overwhelmed.
- ☞ Balances the three doshas (vata, pitta, kapha); helps improve digestive fire as well as lung capacity.
- ☞ Improves respiratory functions and gastric health. Users claim relief from constipation.
- ☞ Supports gall bladder and liver functioning. Individuals practising the mudra have credited it with aiding in the management of diabetes.

- Calms the mind and improves the sleep cycle.
- Helps find peace and calm amidst emotional conflicts.

BRONCHIAL MUDRA

This mudra is effective in treating conditions such as asthma, bronchitis, allergies and other respiratory symptoms caused by pollution. It helps improve lung function and promotes deep, calm breathing. When respiration is shallow and improper, people with bronchial issues experience loneliness and weakness. Bronchial Mudra helps overcome all these.

Hand Formation:

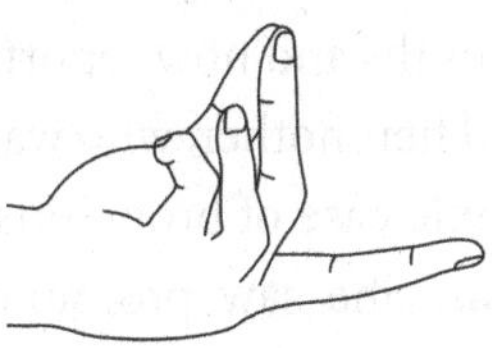

- Bring the tip of the little finger to the base of the thumb.
- Place the ring finger on the upper joint of the thumb.
- Touch the tip of the middle finger to the tip of the thumb.
- Keep the index finger straight.
- Both hands should assume the same gesture.
- During severe asthma attacks, in addition to what has been prescribed by your healthcare professional, hold this mudra for five minutes, followed by the Asthma Mudra for another five. This can be repeated several times a day during asthma attacks.

Benefits:

- Improves the respiratory function. Reported to be good for asthma, bronchitis, allergies and respiratory disorders caused by pollution.

- Promotes deeper, more effective breathing. Reduces wheezing and coughing.
- Many have indicated using the mudra to help overcome sadness, depression and loneliness.
- Helps you find inner strength and balances the five elements.
- Oxygen intake increases as wind pipes open up; bronchial tubes are dilated.

ASTHMA MUDRA

Asthmatic conditions can be triggered by allergic conditions, environmental issues or emotional situations. In all these cases, this mudra can be of aid.

An acquaintance with long-standing asthma held this mudra for forty-five minutes daily for over two months and now reports full recovery. Another woman I know asked her mother, who was over seventy-five years old and had a chronic case of bronchitis, to try the Bronchial and Asthma Mudras. She saw profound results: the chest and nose blocks were instantly better, and the old lady was reported to be in a happy and calm state of mind after just one sitting.

Hand Formation:

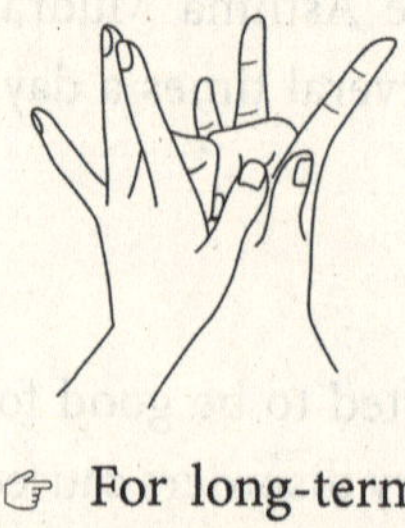

- Hold both hands at the chest level.
- Bend the upper halves of the middle fingers and press the finger nails against each other.
- Keep all the other fingers extended and slightly apart.
- For long-term treatment, this mudra should be held for fifteen to twenty minutes daily for forty-five days.

Benefits:

- ☞ It helps clear the nadis and removes blockages to the lungs.
- ☞ Helps in balancing vata and kapha doshas. These imbalances restrict the flow of prana to the lungs, leading to difficulty in breathing.
- ☞ This mudra activates the Akasha Tatva; it relaxes the bronchial tubes, expands the lungs, clears blockages and releases toxins.
- ☞ Reported to help reduce wheezing and coughing.
- ☞ Balances the flow of energy in the body, thus having a calming effect on the entire system.

As you practise this mudra, visualise the lungs expanding and filling up with fresh air.

MUDRA FOR IRREGULAR HEART PALPITATIONS

For a normal adult, the resting heart rate could be between sixty to hundred beats per minute. When it goes below sixty (bradycardia) or above hundred (tachycardia), it indicates a need for attention.

Hand Formation:

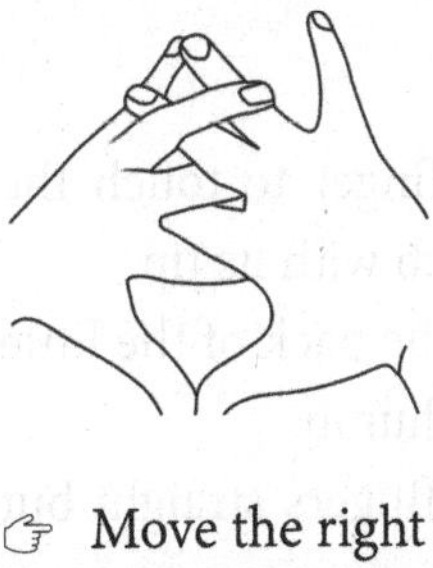

- ☞ Bring both the hands together, palms facing downward.
- ☞ The pads of both thumbs should touch each other.
- ☞ Slip the right index finger between the left index and middle fingers, such that it is below the latter.
- ☞ Move the right middle finger below the left ring finger and bring it in contact with the left little finger.
- ☞ Bring the right ring finger across the left middle finger and below the left ring finger so that it touches the tip of the left little finger.

☞ The right little finger should remain free.

Benefits:

☞ Testimonials have indicated that it can reduce heart palpitations and control irregular heartbeat.

☞ Reported to regulate weakness and dizziness due to irregular heartbeat.

JALODHARA NASHAKA MUDRA

This mudra is designed to promote balance in the body's water element and address various health issues related to fluid retention and hydration. The term jalodhara translates to water in the stomach, and nashaka means to finish, or to eliminate, indicating the mudra's purpose in managing water-related imbalances.

The Jalodhara Nashaka Mudra is highly effective for a runny nose. Many people have reported that after practising it before bed, they woke up to find their symptoms had subsided. While practising the mudra, visualise excess water being released from your body. Imagine achieving your goals and experiencing joy and freedom.

Hand Formation:

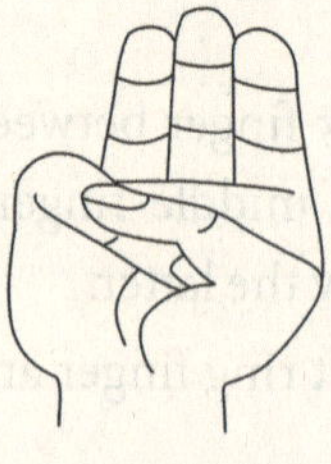

☞ Bend the little finger to touch the base of the thumb with its tip.

☞ Press down on the back of the little finger with the thumb.

☞ Keep the other fingers straight but relaxed.

Rajendar Menen (2019) finds this mudra good to get rid of excess mucous that collects in the lungs and the stomach (p. 66).

Excessive mucous leads to overstimulation of the nerves, inner tensions, overstraining, and restlessness of the body and mind.

Benefits:

- Could help to control swelling and water retention in the body.
- Testimonials claim that there have been cases where it has cured elephantiasis.
- It is good for excessive urination, salivation, watery eyes, runny nose and hyperacidity.
- Helps with pleurisy.
- It is suggested to aid with menstrual health. There have been cases where the menstrual cycle could be postponed by practising the mudra for fifteen minutes daily during the three days leading up to the expected date.

KUBERA MUDRA

Kubera is the god of wealth. This mudra brings abundance and financial prosperity to those who practise it. Here, the intensity is more important than the length of time involved. This mudra is a combination of three mudras—Vyana Mudra, Surya Mudra and Jalodhara Nashaka Mudra. The mudra enables you to align your energy with the energy of abundance, as all five elements are activated.

Kubera Mudra is immensely useful in dissolving phlegm accumulated in the frontal sinuses. Unaware of its immediate effects, an acquaintance tried holding this mudra while at work. She later contacted me, surprised that even after a brief period of practice, she found herself having to frequently clear her nose.

Hand Formation:

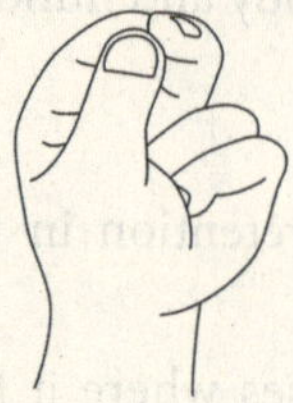

- ☞ Touch the ring and little fingers to the base of the thumb.
- ☞ Lightly touch the tips of index finger, middle finger and thumb together.

Benefits:

- ☞ Boosts energy levels and enhances blood circulation.
- ☞ Practitioners of the mudra have claimed that it helps open up the frontal sinuses, thereby decongesting and cleaning them.
- ☞ Reported to help with clearing a blocked nose, alleviating heaviness in the head and with headache due to sinus.
- ☞ Kubera Mudra gives us the courage to make projects succeed; the energy is concentrated and you can direct it as you wish.
- ☞ Strengthens your resolve and provides the confidence and calmness of mind to move ahead.
- ☞ Generates positive thoughts, and helps in attaining goals and fulfilling wishes.

Hold the mudra for thirty seconds and visualise your wishes being fulfilled. Express gratitude. Make your wish statement in advance and keep it short. Then keep holding the mudra for at least fifteen minutes. Ideally, the duration should be increased gradually over time. To attain the best results for financial stability, practise this mudra for forty-five minutes daily for twenty-one days. However, this mudra does not guarantee financial stability; it simply changes the practitioner's mindset and attracts positivity.

Contraindications:

- ☞ It may aggravate pain or cause additional strain for those with arthritis, wrist injury and carpal tunnel syndrome.

- This mudra aggravates vata, and therefore those exhibiting excess vata symptoms, like dizziness, poor circulation or dryness, should avoid its practice. Both the Air and Space elements are enhanced here, which may aggravate certain symptoms.

LINGA MUDRA

Linga Mudra is a hand gesture that symbolises the integration of the masculine and feminine energies. Linga means phallus or symbol in Sanskrit, referring to the upright thumb that resembles a phallus. The interlocked fingers form an oval shape at the base, representing the feminine energy, or shakti. The practice of this mudra must be discontinued once the problem is resolved. Those with hyperacidity, ulcers or high fever should not practise this mudra.

Hand Formation:

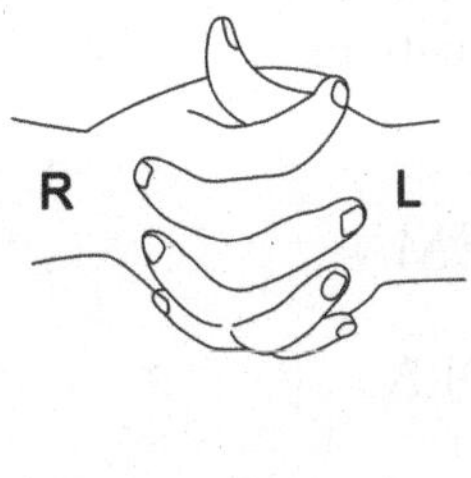

- Interlock the fingers of both hands by weaving them together.
- Raise the left-hand thumb.
- Wrap the index finger and thumb of the right hand around the left-hand thumb.

Benefits:

- Stimulates the immune system. It is reported to increase the body's resistance to cold, cough and chest infections.
- Loosens the mucus collected in the lungs.
- Imbalances of kapha are corrected.

- Beneficial for respiratory complaints caused by changes in the weather.
- It can help reduce mild fevers.
- Individuals have reported that it enhances digestive power and burns the excess fat in the body.
- Helps in restoring the navel centre to its proper position. To do this, hold the mudra and stand with your feet shoulder-width apart. Then, with a jerk, bring your hands down. Repeat the mudra ten to fifteen times.

Contraindications:

- Linga Mudra increases heat in the body, so it should be practised for a maximum of fifteen minutes, except when congestion is severe. In that case, hold it for thirty minutes, followed by Prana Mudra for ten minutes.
- As this mudra generates heat, it can easily make you dehydrated. You will need to drink plenty of water before and after holding this mudra.
- The mudra should not be used to manage high fevers. It may cause harmful effects if used in such situations.

DIGESTIVE SYSTEM

JALA VRUDDHI MUDRA

Jala Vruddhi Mudra is a powerful practice for enhancing the Water element in the body. By incorporating this mudra into your daily routine, you can experience its numerous physical, emotional and spiritual benefits. The practice of this mudra must be discontinued once the problem is resolved.

Hand Formation:

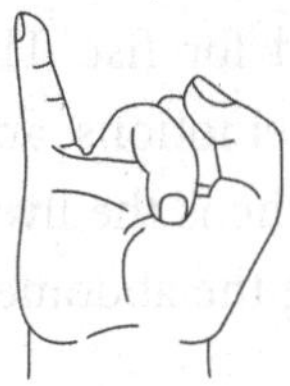

- Fold the index, middle and ring fingers into the palm.
- Press them lightly with the thumb.
- The little finger remains straight, which enhances the Jala Tatva.

Benefits:

- Reported to promote regular urination and helps eliminate toxins through urine.
- Mudra practitioners have claimed it is helpful in cases of dehydration, diarrhoea and excessive dry skin.

MATANGI MUDRA

This is a therapeutic mudra that helps practitoners transcend the physical nature of our lives. One should hold the mudra while focusing on the Anahata Chakra.

Hand Formation:

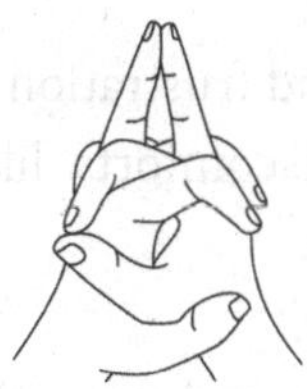

- Bring both the hands together.
- Interlace all the fingers.
- Extend the middle fingers, pressing them against each other.

Benefits:

- Many users claim that it helps alleviate stomach ailments.
- Good for overall health of the abdominal organs.
- Enhances immunity by strengthening the lymphatic system.
- Has a calming effect on the nervous system.
- Reported to be useful for managing fistulas.

MUSHTI MUDRA

The term mushti comes from the Sanskrit word for fist. The fist gesture is effective for managing negative emotions and promoting overall well-being. This mudra strengthens the liver, stomach, pancreas and intestines, thereby keeping the abdomen healthy.

When holding this mudra, reflect on the emotions to be released and visualise them dissipating with every exhalation.

Hand Formation:

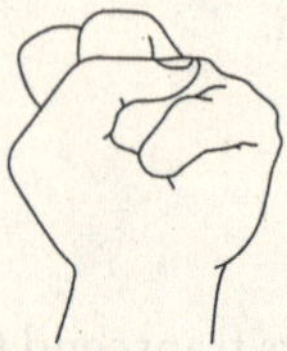

- Clench your fingers to form a fist.
- Stretch the thumb across the index and middle fingers to press down on the ring finger.
- Keep the fist firm but relaxed.

Benefits:

- As the four fingers are pressed by the thumb, it is a combination of Vayu, Shoonya, Surya and Jalodhara Nashaka Mudras, which means all these elements are decreased.
- Helps with feelings of depression, irritation and frustration.
- Reported to aid in relief from physical discomforts like shivering, excess phlegm, inertia and lethargy.
- Reduces tingling in different parts of the body.
- Encourages a positive flow of energy to the liver and stomach.
- Practitioners have mentioned it reduces blood pressure.

PITTA ENERGISING MUDRA

This mudra, as the name suggests, is meant to help people overcome depression and navigate dilemmas. It helps them see the world from a different perspective. Often, we get stuck in repetitive thoughts—much like how an individual who, at the loss of a dear one, withdraws inward, unable to cope with the situation. Such circumstances can be managed by balancing the pitta energy.

Hand Formation:

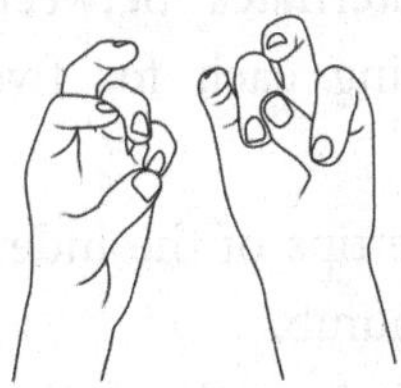

- On the right hand, place the index finger at the first joint of the thumb.
- Place the thumb at the side of the ring finger, beside the nail.
- The left hand is in Jala Mudra—thumb touching the little finger.
- Hold this mudra for three to five minutes, thrice a day.

Benefit:

- The fire element is revitalised and hence reduces negative thoughts, provides motivation and helping one overcome sadness.

POOSHANA MUDRA

The word pooshan, or pushan, is derived from the Sanskrit word pus which means to nourish, protect and guide. Pushan is a Vedic solar deity associated with the sun's nourishing quality and hence referred to as the god of nourishment. This mudra helps maintain the digestive fire essential for better absorption of nutrients from the food we intake. In acute cases of indigestion, bloating, etc., holding this mudra for forty-five minutes in addition to following your healthcare professional's advice may prove beneficial.

While holding the Pooshana Mudra, visualise your digestive system working efficiently, promoting health and vitality.

Hand Formation:

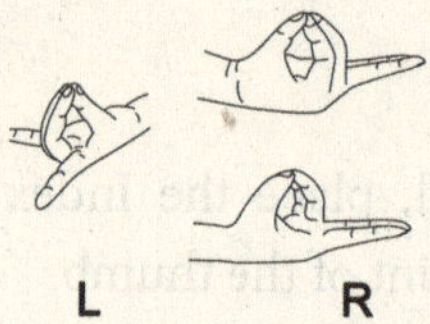

- The left hand is in Apana Mudra—join the finger-tips of the middle and ring fingers with the tip of the thumb.
- The right-hand alternates between two mudras, holding each for five minutes:
  - First, the hand in is Vyana Mudra—the tips of the index and middle fingers touch the tip of the thumb.
  - After five minutes, change to Prana Mudra—the tips of ring and little fingers touch the tip of the thumb.

Benefits:

- Equilibrium of Agni Tatva relaxes the solar plexus.
- Helps with nourishment, absorption of food and building immunity, while also facilitating elimination.
- Helps in better absorption of prana from the air we breathe; also facilitates release of CO_2 from the lungs.
- Practitioners of the mudra have observed that it provides relief from acute nausea, flatulence, heaviness after a meal and seasickness.
- Improves overall immunity and general health.

PRANA VAYU MUDRA

This is a combination of two mudras—Prana Mudra and Vayu Mudra.

Hand Formation:

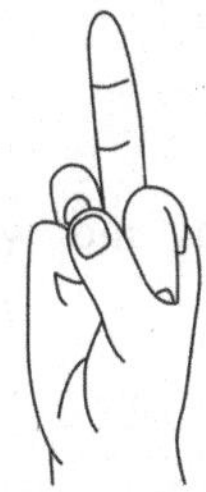

- Hold the Vayu Mudra—touch the index finger to the base of the thumb.
- Lightly press down on the index finger with the thumb.
- Form the Prana Mudra by touching the tips of little and ring fingers with the thumb pad.
- Keep the middle finger straight.

Benefits:

- Relaxes the heart and improves respiratory health.
- Reported to regulate blood pressure.
- According to various testimonials, it helps in acute cases of bloody, sticky or loose motion.
- Activates the parasympathetic nervous system. Many who employ the mudra have indicated that it is beneficial for insomnia, depression and anxiety.

RUDRA MUDRA

Rudra is the presiding deity in Manipura Chakra, the symbol of Fire. This mudra activates the Manipura Chakra.

Hand Formation:

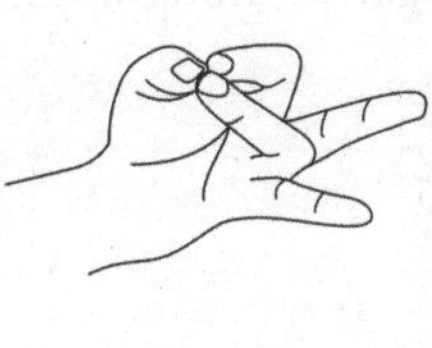

- Lightly touch the tips of the thumb, index finger and ring finger together.
- Keep the other two fingers straight but relaxed.

Benefits:

- Activates the Manipura Chakra; helps maintain the health of the abdominal organs.
- Prithvi Tatva is enhanced, resulting in increased energy in the brain.
- Enhances the pitta in the navel.
- Improves digestion.
- Boosts self-confidence.
- Helps recover from lethargy, laziness and may aid with depression.

SUCHI MUDRA

Suchi Mudra, also known as the Needle Mudra, helps stimulate and balance the doshas while also aiding in kundalini awakening.

Hand Formation:

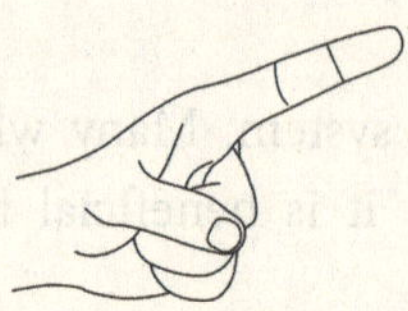

- Curl in the little, ring and middle fingers while keeping your index finger extended.
- Press the thumb over the curled fingers; stretch the thumb as far as possible over the curled fingers.

- Ideally, practise the mudra on an empty stomach

Benefits:

- Reported to aid with constipation.
- Gives control over the mind; supresses negative thoughts and emotions.
- Sharpens focus and enhances memory.
- Stabilises the mind and body.

ENDOCRINE SYSTEM

KANISHTA MUDRA

The word kanishta in Sanskrit typically refers to the smallest or youngest, often associated with the little finger or something of the least importance. The little finger is generally associated with the element of Water and represents fluidity, communication and emotional expression.

A participant who repeated the course with me twice reached out recently narrating how, after three decades, her high blood pressure was finally brought under control within a few days of practising this mudra.

Hand Formation:

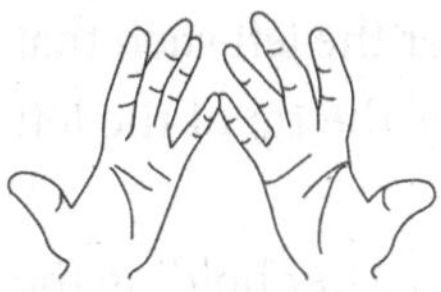

- Lightly touch the tips of the two little fingers together, palms facing upward.
- Keep the other fingers stretched out.
- Hold the position at the heart centre.

Benefits:

- Practitioners report that the mudra improves blood flow and regulates blood pressure.
- As the blood pressure is regulated, it brings calmness and makes one stress-free.
- Improves bowel health. Practitioners have claimed that it relieves constipation.
- Increases bone density; improves the skeletal structure of the body.

SHANKHA MUDRA

This mudra resembles a conch and is hence named Shankha Mudra. A conch is blown for all auspicious occasions and its waves of positive energy spread far and wide. This mudra too has numerous benefits. A patient reported that her thyroid levels were back to normal within forty-five days of practising this mudra for twenty minutes daily.

Hand Formation:

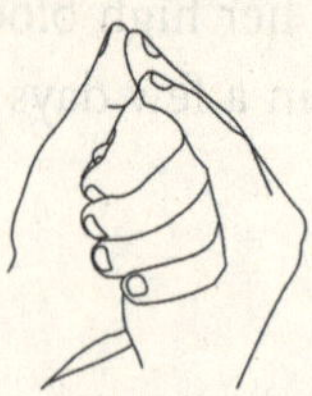

- Bring the pad of the right thumb to the base of the left thumb.
- Wrap the remaining four fingers of the left hand over the right thumb.
- Lay the four fingers of the right hand over the left such that the tip of the right middle finger touches the tip of the left thumb.
- Reverse hand positions after ten minutes. After holding the mudra on each hand, circle the base of both thumbs with the index finger and thumb of the opposite hand a few times, both clockwise and anti-clockwise.

Benefits:

- Holding the thumb of one hand by the fingers of the other suppresses the Fire element in the body; touching the middle finger with the thumb balances the Ether element. Thus, more space is created within the body, thereby stimulating assimilation and digestion processes.
- The inner fingers form a spiral, like the coil of the human digestive system. Therefore, Shankha Mudra calms the excessive digestive fires that cause constipation and ulcers.

- Activates the Vishuddha Chakra and consequently, the vocal cords; improves confidence in speaking in front of others.
- Improves the functioning of the larynx; in some case, it may help with managing stammering and stuttering disorders.
- Increases appetite by stimulating the digestive system.
- Practised along with the OM chanting, it rejuvenates the 72,000 nadis. The vibration thus produced stimulates the thyroid glands that secrete thyroxine and triiodothyronine hormones. Reports suggest that it can help with hypothyroidism and associated problems.
- In many users of the mudra, it has aided with rashes, dry skin and allergies. Skin dryness occurs when the Fire element is high; this mudra subdues it.
- May result in an increase in height in growing children; rejuvenates the entire body.
- Good for kidneys.
- People practising this mudra have mentioned that it provides relief from tonsillitis, throat infections and allergies caused by dust and smoke.
- There are situations where it has helped in the recovery of speech after a paralytic attack.
- Has a calming effect and removes negativities.

SHOONYA MUDRA

Shoonya means emptiness or void. This mudra helps channel the Akasha Tatva in the body. Many mudra practitioners hold this mudra when on a flight to prevent blocked ears and ear pain. It cannot heal congenital defects.

Hand Formation:

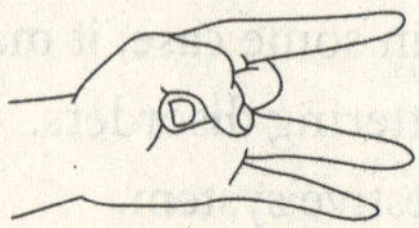

☞ Gently press the middle finger into the palm using the thumb.

☞ Keep all the other fingers straight but relaxed.

Benefits:

☞ Prevents weakness and reduces numbness in the body.

☞ Good for short-tempered people; brings peace, tranquillity and calmness.

☞ Enhances auditory health.

☞ Reduces excessive sweating of the palms.

☞ Improves blood circulation.

☞ Due to frequent changes in cabin air pressure during flight landing or take off, the eustachian tubes can be blocked or obstructed, preventing the middle ear pressure from being equalised. The resultant vacuum sucks the eardrum inward, hindering its ability to vibrate naturally. This causes pain and discomfort, which can be minimised by holding the mudra just before take-off or landing.

☞ Reported to aid with vertigo; once vertigo has been cured, Akasha Mudra should be performed daily for fifteen minutes to avoid recurrence.

USHAS MUDRA

This mudra symbolises new beginnings and the awakening of the consciousness. The term ushas means dawn in Sanskrit, and this mudra is associated with the Goddess Ushas, who represents light and the arrival of a new day.

Hand Formation:

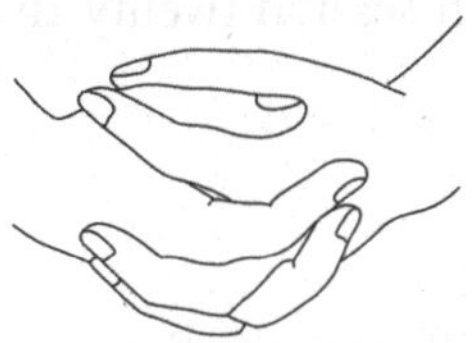

- Interlace your fingers, ensuring that the palms are facing inward.
- For men: place the right thumb on top of the left thumb and apply gentle pressure.
- For women: place the left thumb on top of the right thumb, with the right thumb positioned between the left thumb and index finger.
- While holding the mudra, visualise it is dawn—the beginning of the positive changes you want in life.

Benefits:

- Promotes hormonal health. There are reports that it is beneficial for PCOD and thyroid health.
- Supports menstrual health.
- Activates the Swadhisthana Chakra and enhances creativity.
- As a meditative mudra that embodies the qualities of the sun, it revitalises life.
- Provides inner nourishment and calm.
- It activates the Agni Tatva, aiding in digestion, purification and transformation. The mudra provides internal warmth.
- Practitioners have attested to gaining relief from heartburn and hyperacidity.

MUSCULOSKELETAL DISORDERS

KEELA MUDRA

Holding this mudra helps balance the space between the cartilage and the joint muscles. It is particularly good for joint pains. So, this mudra should be used in conjunction with Vayu Mudra and

Prana Mudra. For acute pain, the Keela Mudra should be held six times a day for eight minutes each, each session twenty-five minutes apart.

Hand Formation:

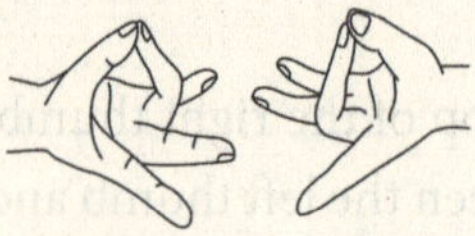

- Both hands in different positions.
- Hold the Akasha Mudra with the left hand—the tips of middle finger and thumb come into light contact.
- Hold the Prithvi Mudra with the right hand—the tips of the ring finger and thumb come into light contact.

Benefits:

- Can enhance calcium levels.
- Alleviates fatigue in the elbows after long hours at the computer.
- Various users of this mudra have claimed that it provides relief from hip and knee pain caused by arthritis.
- Can provide relief from customary aches after hiking or climbing downhill.

KATI MUDRA (SPINE MUDRA OR MERUDANDA MUDRA)

The Sanskrit term kati refers to the waist or lower back. This mudra focuses on the lumbar and pelvic region. It is particularly beneficial for improving posture, relieving lower back pain and enhancing energy flow in the body.

When holding the Kati Mudra, visualise energy flowing through the lower back and healing the area.

Hand Formation:

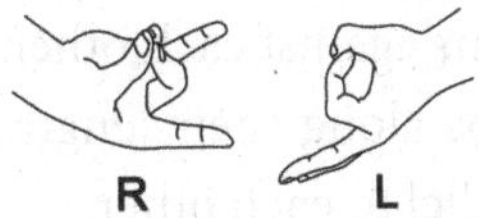

- On the right hand, touch the tips of the middle and little fingers to the tip of the thumb.
- Keep the other two fingers straight but relaxed.
- On the left hand, the index finger is slightly bent to touch the first joint of the thumb.
- Bend the thumb over the tip of the index finger.
- Keep the other fingers straight but relaxed.

Benefits:

- Helps alleviate tension and discomfort in the lower back, promoting relaxation and a better posture.
- Aids in bringing relief from all types of physical strain—due to household work, gardening or long hours working at the desk.
- Helps with mental strain and fears.
- Balances the Mooladhara Chakra and supports digestive health.
- Holding the mudra for thirty minutes, followed by the Prana Mudra for ten, is proposed to support the healing of a slipped disc.

SAHAJA SHANKHA MUDRA

The word sahaja in Sanskrit means ease, so this literally translates to simplified Shankha Mudra. The mudra helps heal several ailments and has a calming effect. It should ideally be practised early in the morning.

Hand Formation:

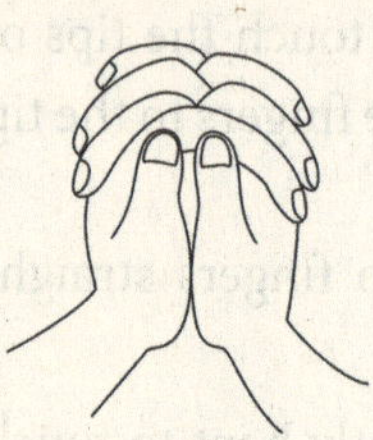

☞ Interlock the fingers of both hands, pressing the palms against each other.

☞ Join both thumbs along their length, laying them parallel to each other.

☞ Press down on the index finger of the right hand.

Benefits:

☞ Activates the ten major nerve channels, including the Sushumna, Ida and Pingala Nadis.

☞ Enhanced alertness.

☞ Mudra practitioners are known to use it to relieve ailments related to the anus, including piles.

☞ A strengthened spinal cord and increased flexibility in the vertebral column. It is claimed to help with a bulging disc.

☞ Improves speech and digestion.

☞ Beneficial for reproductive issues.

GYNAECOLOGICAL ISSUES

MAHATRIKA MUDRA

Mahatrika, or 'the great triangle', is a healing mudra particularly beneficial for the pelvic region. In this mudra, the little fingers touch each other, balancing the Jala Tatva. The mudra should be held for seven to eight minutes, thrice a day.

Hand Formation:

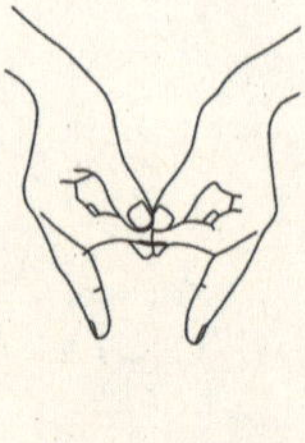

☞ Palms facing each other, extend the little fingers so that the tips touch.

☞ Bring the thumbs and index fingers of both hands together.

- Keep the ring and middle fingers straight but relaxed.
- Bend the wrists slightly so that the fingers point downward.

Benefits:

- As the mudra governs the pelvic region, it promotes menstrual and reproductive health.
- Many women who practise the mudra claim that it helps manage menopausal symptoms.
- Effective for prostate, urinary and bladder health.
- Users of this mudra indicate that it provides relief from constipation and works as a remedy for stomach cramps.
- There are testimonials that suggest that it can be an aid to support recovery from hernia and haemorrhoids.
- Helps remove emotional blockages.

SHAKTI MUDRA

As the name suggests, this mudra personifies the goddess of strength, Shakti, and thus provides power and strength. When the little and ring fingers are joined together, the Prithvi Tatva and Jala Tatva are balanced, correcting the kapha imbalance. Fingers pointing downward help activate the Apana Vayu, further aiding the release of toxins within us.

Hand Formation:

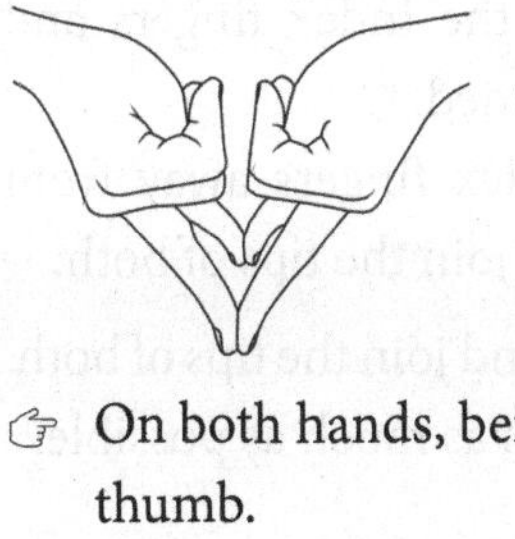

- Join the tips of the little and ring fingers to the corresponding fingers of the other hand.
- On both hands, fold the thumb into the palm.
- On both hands, bend the index and middle fingers over the thumb.

- Tilt the wrists downward.

Benefits:

- Improves the functioning of the urinary and reproductive systems.
- The Mooladhara and Swadhisthana Chakras are balanced, thereby making one feel grounded while also developing the ability to go with the flow.
- Helps you become more flexible and adaptive in life.
- Soothes the nervous system and calms the mind.
- Aids in improving the sleep cycle.

UTTARA BODHI/YONI MUDRA

The word uttara in Sanskrit means upward or highest, and bodhi means enlightenment. This mudra of enlightenment encourages and strengthens inhalation and the absorption of oxygen. It refreshes and revitalises the body while also strengthening the energy of the lungs, intestines and heart.

Interestingly, this mudra is known to be used before an important event, such as before signing an agreement, attending a conference, etc.

Hand Formation:

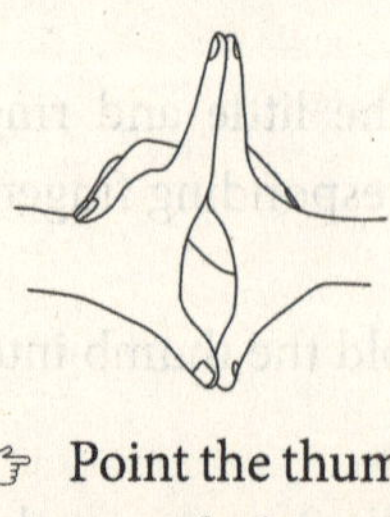

- Interlock all the fingers together, leaving only the index fingers and thumbs extended.
- Point the index fingers away from the body and join the tips of both.
- Point the thumbs towards the body and join the tips of both.
- Stretch the index fingers and thumbs as much as possible.

- Keep your hands close to the navel, or the Swadhisthana chakra.

Benefits:

- Supports menstrual health. Many women have testified that it helps relieve cramps, pains, menopausal symptoms, heavy or scanty menstrual flow, as well as irritation and anger during the menstrual cycle.
- It is believed to assist in the management of PCOD and fibroids.
- For menopausal issues, it is suggested that you hold the Uttara Bodhi Mudra for ten minutes, followed by the Prana Mudra for another ten.
- Strengthens the nervous system; alleviates stress and improves concentration.
- Stimulates the Manipura Chakra, thereby boosting confidence.
- Facilitates meditation and improves cardiovascular health.

Contraindication:

- This mudra generates heat and should therefore be discontinued immediately once the problem is resolved.

OTHER CURATIVE MUDRAS

ADI MUDRA

Adi Mudra balances Udana Vayu, stimulating both Prana and Udana. For hand formation and benefits, refer to Chapter Six.

For help with fear and anxiety, follow the process:

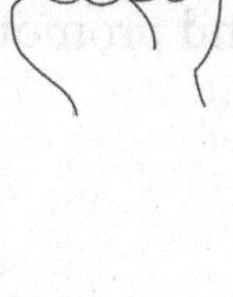

- Hold the hands in Adi Mudra.
- Inhale and hold the breath.
- Chant OM seven times while holding the breath.

☞ Exhale while releasing fears, worries and anxieties.

ADITI MUDRA

The word aditi in Sanskrit is often associated with the concept of infinity, or boundlessness. Aditi is considered the mother of all gods and therefore symbolises nurturing and protection. Aditi Mudra enhances the Earth element.

Hand Formation:

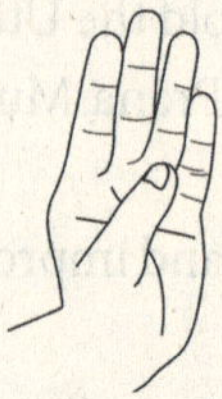

☞ Lightly bring the pad of the thumb to the base of the ring finger (the ring finger represents the Earth element).

☞ Keep the other fingers straight but relaxed.

Benefits:

☞ It is said by mudra instructors that with a minimum of fifty minutes of practice per day, this mudra will help you gain weight.

☞ It is reported to help control sneezing, particularly in those prone to sneezing in the early hours.

☞ Reduces yawning.

☞ Removes toxins from the body.

BHRAMARA MUDRA

The name bhramara comes from the Sanskrit word for bee, symbolising the qualities of hard work and flexibility. Also known as the bee gesture, this is a hand position used in yoga and meditation that can help alleviate allergic reactions and promote overall well-being.

Hand Formation:

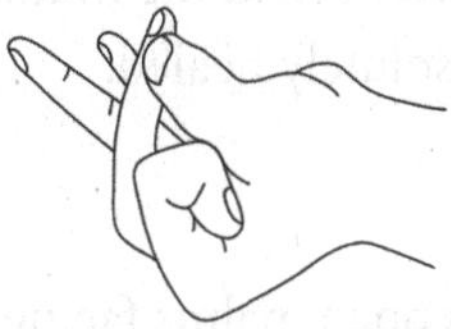

- ☞ Touch the tip of the index finger to the base of the thumb.
- ☞ Lightly touch the tip of the thumb to the side of the middle finger's fingernail.
- ☞ Keep the other two fingers straight but relaxed.

Benefits:

- ☞ Users of the mudra claim that it strengthens the immune system and alleviates allergies.
- ☞ Improves concentration, memory and confidence.
- ☞ Calms the nervous system, promoting a better sleep cycle and reducing stress.
- ☞ Opens up the sinus and nasal passages, aiding those with frequent congestion.
- ☞ Reported to be beneficial for those prone to pollen allergies.
- ☞ Promotes respiratory health. According to practitioners of the mudra, it eases conditions like wheezing, bronchitis and asthma.

FUNGUS MUDRA

This mudra is reported to aid the body in fighting off fungal infections, particularly those affecting the skin and nails. My personal experience with this mudra is worth sharing. I came across this mudra during the course of my research and started using it on myself. I had developed a small infection on my left ankle and despite trying all sorts of allopathic medicines, ointments, home remedies and homeopathy, there was no relief.

The moment I discovered this mudra, I decided to give it a try. I saw results from the third day itself. After I held the mudra thrice a day for fifteen days, the area was absolutely healed.

Hand Formation

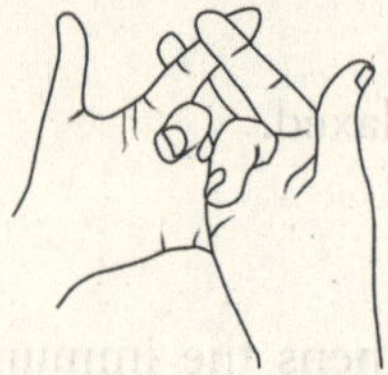

- Hold both hands open, palms facing upward.
- Bend both the middle fingers down.
- Place the right index finger over the left index finger.
- Place the right ring finger behind the left index finger in such a way that the bases of both ring fingers touch.
- Place the little fingers of both hands in such a manner that the bases of both fingers touch.
- Keep the thumbs apart.
- Hold the mudra thrice a day, for five, eight and twelve minutes, respectively.

Benefits:

- Many people who have tried this mudra claim that regular practice of the mudra has helped them overcome fungal infection. In other cases, it is reported to have reduced the discomfort associated with fungal outbreaks.
- Promotes immunity.

HERPES MUDRA

Herpes is caused by a virus, and it can result in unbearable pain and discomfort. It may also lead to fever-like symptoms and cause itching. When holding this mudra, visualise the healing energy flowing through your body, promoting balance and well-being.

Hand Formation:

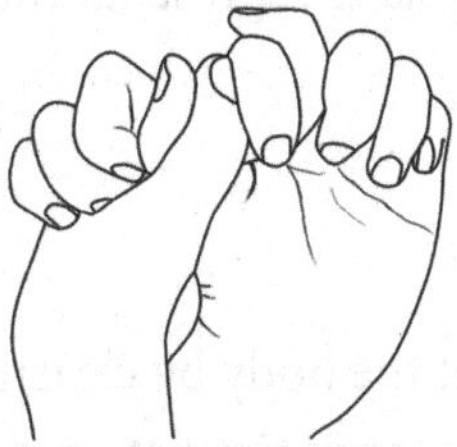

- Place the back of the right palm over the back of the left.
- Lock the index fingers of both hands.
- Bring the pads of both thumbs into contact with each other.

Benefits:

- Individuals who have utilised this mudra state that it helps develop the strength to fight the herpes virus. In addition, they attest that it can also alleviate the pain caused by the infection.
- The mudra is reported to help eliminate skin rashes.
- Promotes emotional balance.

KALI MUDRA

This mudra helps eliminate the unwanted, thereby enabling vitality, fresh energy and positivity to enter the system. In fact, as one moves forward in life, one must learn to release the unwanted, and travel light to make the journey smoother.

Hand Formation:

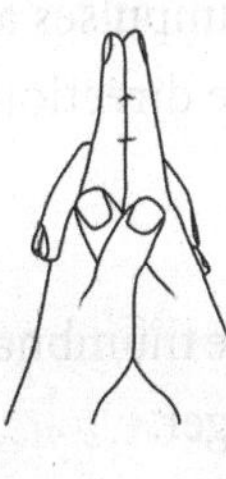

- Palms facing each other, interlock all but the index fingers.
- Extend the index fingers straight and place their tips flat against each other, creating a pointed shape that symbolises the sword of the goddess Kali.

- Cross your thumbs, with the left thumb resting over the right. This positioning is significant, as it represents the balance of energies.
- Hold the mudra at the heart centre.

Benefits:

- Enhances the flow of prana throughout the body by clearing blockages in the nadis. This improved energy circulation can lead to increased vitality and a sense of rejuvenation.
- Aids in physical detoxification, as it stimulates the digestive and respiratory systems.
- Releases muscular tension, particularly in the neck, throat and shoulders.
- By clearing negative thoughts and emotions, it helps improve focus and mental clarity.
- Alleviates stress and anxiety.
- Stimulates the Throat and Crown chakras, enhancing communication and spiritual awareness.
- Boosts metabolism.

KAMAJAYI MUDRA

Kamajayi Mudra is a hand gesture used in yoga and meditation practices to help control and overcome desires or cravings. Kama in Sanskrit means desire, while jayi means to conquer or control. This mudra helps you gain better control over your impulses and inspires you to channel your energy in more positive directions.

Hand Formation:

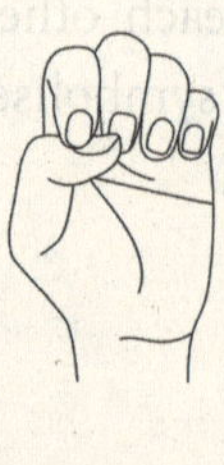

- Press down on the root of the thumbnail with the tip of the index finger.
- Keep the other fingers relaxed and slightly curled.

Benefits:

- ☞ The mudra is reported to help restrain addictions such as overeating, drinking and smoking.
- ☞ Aids in transforming physical energy (ojas) into spiritual energy (tejas).
- ☞ Helps connect with the power within.
- ☞ Boosts immunity.
- ☞ Pressing down on the thumb reduces the excessive fire energy within us, thereby helping us control our anger and shift our focus towards creative pursuits.

KIDNEY MUDRA

The bladder, located in the pelvic cavity, serves as the reservoir for urine, with its size and position varying based on how much it holds. Its key trait is adaptability, as it first collects and then releases. The name of this mudra draws a parallel to this function of the kidneys, stressing the importance of letting go of emotions—just as a vessel must be emptied before it can be refilled. Kidneys manage the electrolyte balance within the body by regulating sodium concentration in the blood. They clean and detoxify the body to maintain the balance of nutrients. Jala Tatva enhances kidney function.

Hand Formation:

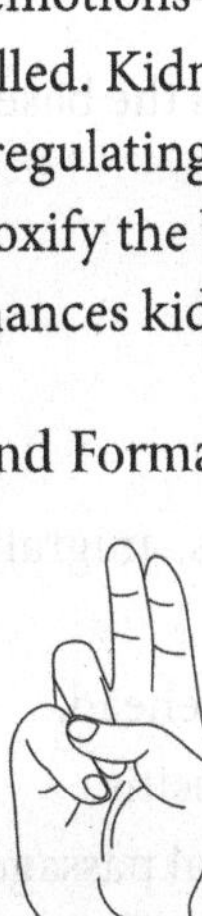

- ☞ Bring the tips of the ring and little fingers to the base of the thumb.
- ☞ Lightly press down on these two fingers with the thumb, keeping the other fingers straight.

Benefits:

- ☞ Removes excess water from the body and promotes kidney function.
- ☞ Controls excessive mucus production.
- ☞ Helps control a runny nose.
- ☞ Improves the health of the larynx and the respiratory system.
- ☞ It is reported to help cure hyperacidity and diarrhoea.

MAHA SHIRSHA MUDRA

Known as the 'gesture of the great head', this mudra promotes mental clarity and alleviates various ailments. It governs the eye sockets and nasal passages, areas associated with headaches or a sense of heaviness in the head.

Hand Formation:

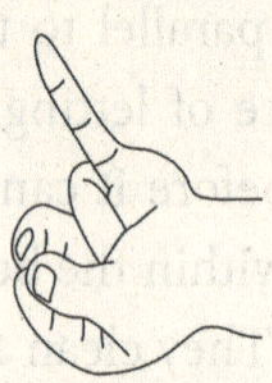

- ☞ Bring the tips of the thumb, index and middle fingers together, pointing upward.
- ☞ Curl the ring finger towards the base of the thumb and rest it there.
- ☞ Extend the little finger towards the ceiling.

Benefits:

- ☞ It is claimed to provide relief from headaches, migraines, tension and sinus congestion.
- ☞ Helps with congestion in the eye sockets and forehead.
- ☞ Reduces facial pain caused by congestion or sinusitis.
- ☞ Decreases the pressure on the eyes, ears and nasal passages.
- ☞ Helps reduce acute stress and relaxes the muscles around the neck.

Precautions:

- Maintain a comfortable position to avoid physical strain.
- Begin with three to five minutes of practice to avoid overstimulation.
- If you experience acute pain in the hands, stop holding the mudra.

PANKAJA (LOTUS) MUDRA

The term pankaja is derived from Sanskrit, panka meaning mud, or clay, and ja meaning born from. Thus, the mudra symbolises the lotus that blooms beautifully despite growing in muddy waters, representing purity and spiritual awakening.

This mudra tells us to live like the lotus flower—rooted in the mud yet rising above it, untouched by the water surrounding it. Just as water droplets are not absorbed by the lotus, the mudra inspires us to remain unattached. It also reminds us that where you come from does not define you. While holding the mudra, visualise a lotus flower blooming within you, representing purity.

Hand Formation:

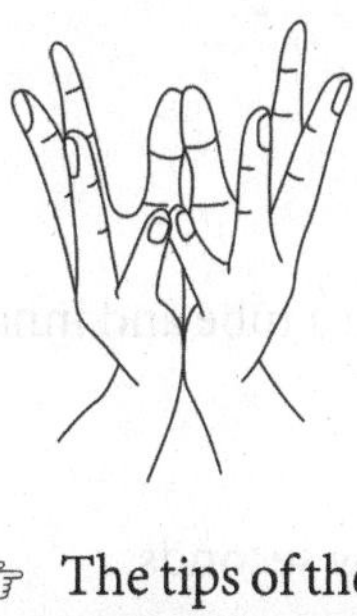

- Bring both hands together in front of the chest at the heart centre, palms facing each other.
- Extend your fingers outward while keeping the thumbs and little fingers touching, forming a shape similar to a lotus flower.
- The tips of the fingers should be slightly curved, resembling the petals of a lotus.
- With eyes closed, take deep breaths and focus on the energy flowing through the hands.

Benefits:

- Gives you a glowing complexion.
- It is suggested to help alleviate unexplained fevers.
- Cools the body and mind.
- Provides emotional cleansing, easing loneliness and grief.
- Reduces feelings of stress and anxiety.
- As the Anahata Chakra is opened, one experiences joy, love and compassion.
- Supports a better sleep cycle.
- Inspires purity and perseverance.
- Various practitioners have successfully treated ulcers using this mudra.
- During meditation, Pankaja Mudra helps maintain focus.

SHEETALI KUMBHAKA IN APANA MUDRA

Sheetali Kumbhaka is a pranayama technique in yoga that involves inhaling through a rolled tongue and exhaling through the nose. This technique helps balance pitta dosha and has a calming effect on the body and mind. When combined with Apana Mudra, the benefits are multiplied.

Hand Formation:

- Hold the hands in Apana Mudra.
- Extend the tongue outside the mouth.
- Curl the sides of the tongue upward to form a tube and inhale through it.
- Roll the tongue back into the mouth.
- Gulp the air in and hold the breath for a few seconds.
- Gradually release the air through the nose.
- Do this ten times before a meal.

Benefits:

- Users practising the mudra have testified that it reduces cholesterol.
- Cools the body and reduces pitta; improves the digestive system.
- Purifies the blood and improves circulation.
- Eliminates toxins.
- Reports from mudra practitioners indicate that it can be effectively wielded to help get rid of addictions.
- It can help with fever and dehydration.

Contraindications:

- Should be avoided by those with kapha disorders like cough, phlegm, sinusitis or asthma.
- Should not be practised in cool climates or in winters.

SURABHI MUDRA AND VARIATIONS

The name Surabhi is derived from a divine cow in Hindu mythology, symbolising abundance and revered for the ability to grant wishes. Also known as Kamadhenu Mudra, it enhances creativity. In spiritual terms, it means to transcend and attain freedom from all desires. One becomes content and has no further desires to be fulfilled. This can help you overcome the barriers in your life, particularly if they are self-imposed. Acharya Keshav Dev calls this mudra the mother of all mudras.

Hand Formation (Surabhi Mudra):

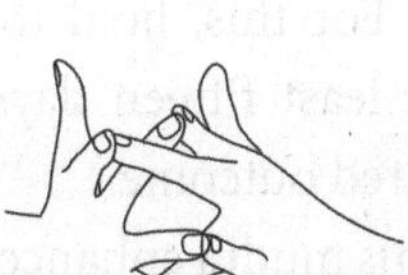

- Bring both hands together in a namaste gesture (palms pressed together, fingers pointing upward) at the heart centre.
- Connect the tip of the ring finger of the right hand to the tip of the little finger of the left hand.

- Connect the tip of the ring finger of the left hand to the tip of the little finger of the right hand.
- Touch the middle fingers of both hands to the index fingers of the opposite hands.
- Extend the thumbs away from the other fingers, keeping them separate and pointing towards you.
- Place the hands between the thighs with the palms facing up.
- Hold the mudra while focusing on your breath and visualising your desires or intentions.

Benefits:

- Activates Jala and Prithvi Tatvas, thereby reducing the pitta dosha.
- Practitioners of the mudra have successfully used it to combat rheumatism.
- At the physical level, it enhances the sense of hearing.
- Improves memory and strengthens concentration power.
- Mudra users have claimed it alleviates gas and acidity.
- Promotes the health of the hormonal and glandular systems, including the adrenaline, pituitary, pineal and thyroid glands.
- Stimulates Manipura Chakra and helps balance the elements, particularly by calming the Fire element.
- Gives you a better understanding of your own talents and latent abilities.
- Balances the tri-doshas.
- Supports creativity.
- It may help in the fulfilment of desires. For this, hold the mudra for ten minutes every day for at least fifteen days, while manifesting and visualising the desired outcome.
- When practised along with Gayatri japa, this mudra enhances one's aura.

VAYU SURABHI MUDRA

Vayu Tatva is enhanced through this mudra and it helps to control the wavering of the mind. The mind is chanchala—Swami Vivekananda (1913) likened the human mind to a monkey, constantly jumping from one branch (thought) to another (p. 66). Thus, when the Vayu Tatva is increased, wavering of the mind is brought under control.

Hand Formation:

- Form the Surabhi Mudra.
- On both hands, touch the pad of the thumb to the base of the index finger.

Benefits:

- Supports consistency and strength of mind.
- Enhances the power of concentration by reducing the wavering of the mind.
- Reported to provide relief from aches and pains.

SHOONYA SURABHI MUDRA

The Akasha Tatva is enhanced in this mudra, allowing one to experience all its benefits. For instance, one experiences avakasha—space and freedom.

Hand Formation:

- Form the Surabhi Mudra.
- On both hands, touch the pad of the thumb to the base of the middle finger.

Benefits:

- ☞ Gives you a calm and peaceful mind, as Akasha Tatva is involved.
- ☞ Prolonged practice of this mudra raises the consciousness and the vibration of the body and mind, and one may even hear the naada brahmam.

PRITHVI SURABHI MUDRA

Here, the Prithvi Tatva is increased, helping to alleviate weakness and support vitality.

Hand Formation:

- ☞ Form the Surabhi Mudra.
- ☞ On both hands, touch the pad of the thumb to the base of the ring finger.

Benefits:

- ☞ Practitioners often report that the mudra improves digestion.
- ☞ It is reported to calm coughs.
- ☞ Alleviates lethargy.

JALA SURABHI MUDRA

It enhances the Jala Tatva, which supports the healing of skin-related issues.

Hand Formation:

- ☞ Form the Surabhi Mudra.
- ☞ On both hands, touch the pad of the thumb to the base of the little finger.

Benefits:

- Helps reduce burning sensations in the body.
- Reduces excessive heat in the body.

The Surabhi Mudra and its variations should be performed for a maximum of five to eight minutes.

CHAPTER 9

Mudras for Brain Revitalisation and Meditation

While the desire to make life materialistically comfortable prevails in us over almost every other consideration, the inner consciousness knows that one has to travel beyond the wordly. According to the *Kaivalya Upanishad*, the lower chakras create bondage while the upper chakras are in the status of OM. Swami Muralidharan, in *Kaivalopanishad: The Key to Liberation*, explains that Fire always travels upward. The lower agni represents ego while the upper agni is OM, the pranava, the primordial sound. Constant chanting of OM or always being in the status of OM (a meditative state), can help one elevate to the higher consciousness. To achieve this status, chant OM with some of the mudras mentioned below.

GARUDA MUDRA

Garuda Mudra symbolises the mythical bird Garuda—the vahana that Maha Vishnu rides. It is believed to have control over the Air element. This mudra is associated with strength, power and protection, and is used to invoke the qualities of the eagle, promoting vitality and energy. The hand positions stimulate the pelvic, abdominal and chest regions sequentially. With breath synchronisation, this mudra relaxes and releases tension in these areas.

Hand Formation:

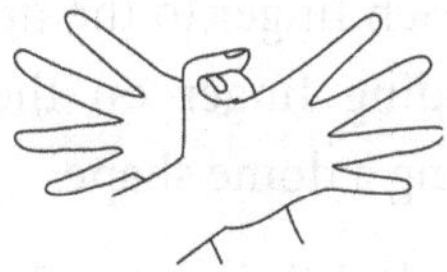

- Raise both hands, palms facing inward.
- Cross the right wrist over the left.
- Interlock the thumbs, hooking the right thumb on the knuckle of the left thumb.
- Extend the remaining fingers.
- Position this gesture over the Anahata (Heart) Chakra.
- This mudra can stimulate different organs depending on its position.

Benefits:

- With the thumbs joined together, there is a burst of energy as Agni Tatva is multiplied.
- Organs for elimination, respiration, blood circulation and digestion are empowered, and function better.
- Immunity is enhanced.
- Aids in keeping your prostate healthy.
- Symbol of strength, protection and freedom.
- Helps control fluctuations of the mind and mood.
- Aids in the removal of fatigue, and generally raises energy levels. For those with high blood pressure, caution is advised.
- Promotes menstrual, reproductive and abdominal health.
- Alleviates exhaustion. Balances Vayu Tatva and vata dosha.

HAKINI MUDRA

Named after the Goddess Hakini, this mudra stimulates the Ajna Chakra. The Ajna Chakra is symbolised by the two-petalled lotus which has many subtle aspects, one of which is Hakini.

Hand Formation:

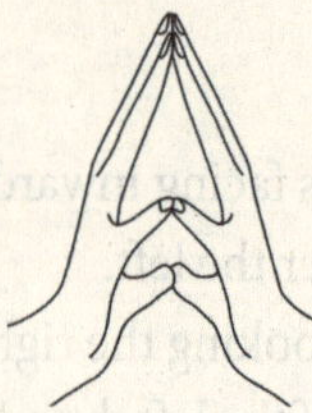

- Bring your palms together at the level of the heart.
- Touch the tip of each finger to the tip of the corresponding finger on the other hand, forming a dome shape.
- Ensure that your fingertips are connected while keeping the palms and fingers slightly apart.

Benefits:

- Hakini Mudra deepens and improves respiration, builds up energy in the lungs, and refreshes and revitalises the brain.
- The right and left hemispheres of the brain are in harmony, and the mind becomes focused.
- It helps improve memory.
- Ensures that the pancha tatvas are in harmony.
- Very helpful in recovery after an illness.
- Practising for longer durations will help the mind become calm. It brings clarity of thought.
- Promotes better sleep patterns.
- It channels the energy required to give us better insight. It also enhances brain function and emotional balance.

BHAIRAVA MUDRA

This mudra symbolises the fierce aspect of Lord Shiva as Bhairava. Bhairava is a powerful manifestation, or avatar, of

Shiva. The word bhairava is derived from the word bhiru, which means terribly fearsome. When holding this mudra, one becomes fearless or overcomes fear. Additionally, it balances energies within the body, enhances the meditation process and promotes overall well-being.

In Bhairava Mudra, the right hand is placed over the left hand. The left hand is governed by the right hemisphere of the brain, often associated with spirituality. When the left hand is positioned below, it directs our actions, bringing them under the influence of the spiritual mind. Conversely, the right hand is connected to the left hemisphere, which is associated with activity. When our actions are guided by the spiritual brain, they align more closely with what is morally right. Additionally, this positioning facilitates the union of Ida and Pingala.

Hand Formation:

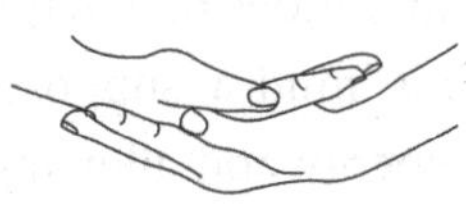

- Place the right hand over the left hand, with both palms facing upward and parallel to the chest.
- Allow the fingers to point in opposite directions, creating a supportive structure.
- Ensure that the thumbs are touching or close together.

Benefits:

- Based on the traits of Bhairava, this mudra has the power to destroy negativity and allow positive characteristics to emerge.
- As we place the palms one upon the other, all centres such as the heart, kidneys, lungs and pancreas are activated along with the spinal nerve points.
- It takes you naturally into a meditative state. One develops a better understanding of the self.

- Makes it easier to connect with the inner consciousness; your presence of mind is strengthened.
- The mudra will help you remain calm amidst adversities. It will promote self-confidence and aid your mental health.

SHIVALINGA MUDRA

The shivalingam symbolises both consciousness and Shiva in constant union with Shakti. The thumb extending upward represents Shiva while the base, or the peetham, is the symbol of Shakti. Among the trinity, Shiva has been entrusted with destruction and transformation. Destruction is not for the purpose of destroying or ending an order but always for paving the way for a new order. It brings about necessary transformation or progress. After all, new beginnings become possible only when the old order is destroyed.

Besides, the upright thumb channels an inflow of energy which is absorbed through the lungs. This mudra supports transformation by ridding the body of old energy and allowing new energy or new inspiration to enter. It also facilitates the process of healing. Thus, one can alleviate fatigue, dissatisfaction and depression.

Hand Formation:

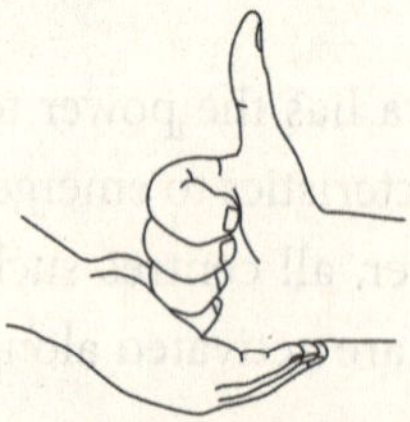

- Hold the left hand at the abdomen level with the palm facing upward.
- Make a loose fist with the right hand and place it over the left palm with the fist facing the body.
- Both elbows rest on the lap.
- The elbows should point outward and forward, parallel to the floor.

Benefits:

- As the thumb is upright, the Fire element is enhanced.
- Enhances will power, and boosts enthusiasm and self-confidence.
- One experiences a heightened sense of vitality as stale energy is replaced with fresh energy.

PRANAMAM MUDRA

Symbolising reverence and gratitude, the mudra is used during prayer in many religions. When all ten fingers touch each other, one's vibrational frequency is enhanced. The mind calms down immediately. This mudra promotes inner peace.

Hand Formation:

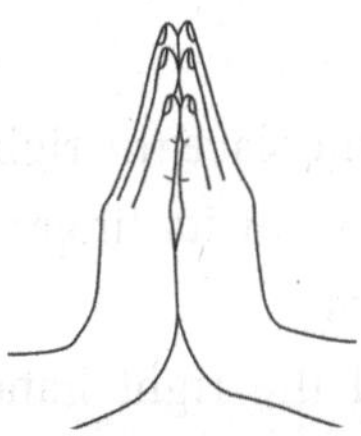

- Bring both palms together in front of the heart centre, similar to a prayer position.
- Elbows should be stretched out so the lungs open up. The thumbs should be placed together at the heart centre.
- Ensure that the fingers are pointing upward and that the palms are pressed together gently.

Benefits:

- Supports harmony, balance, silence, repose and peace.
- Activates and harmonises the coordination of the left and right hemispheres of the brain.
- Enhances concentration and calmness; alleviates anxiety and nerve-related issues.
- Quietens thoughts, stabilises the mind, brings clarity and gives strength.

- The flow of breath through both nostrils is equalised.
- It induces balance of flow in Ida and Pingala.
- Aligns body, mind and spirit, and helps you connect with your inner self.
- Gives you a sense of humility and gratitude.
- This mudra balances the positive side of the body (right, sun, masculine) with the negative side (left, moon, feminine) and this brings harmony into the human system.

NAGA MUDRA

Naga means snake, and snakes are associated with wisdom, shrewdness, cleverness and the ability to navigate through life's obstacles and find solutions to problems. This is a meditative mudra and should ideally be practised in the brahma muhurta.

Hand Formation:

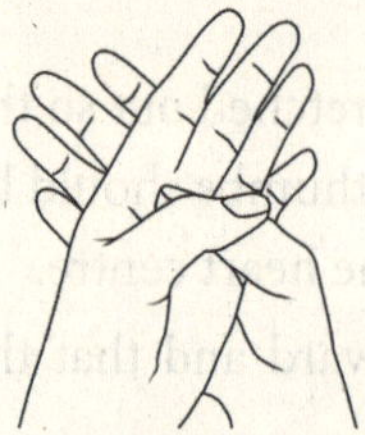

- Open the left palm and place the right thumb across the base of its fingers, perpendicular to them.
- The other fingers of the right hand should wrap around the back of the left.
- Press the thumb of the left hand over the right thumb.
- Keep the other fingers of the left hand straight.
- Place the hands on the lap, close to the navel centre.

Benefits:

- All elements are enhanced, thereby helping in finding solutions to obstacles and problems.
- Creativity and imagination are enhanced.

- You gain clarity of thought.
- While it is a meditative mudra, users of the mudra report that it also helps alleviate issues of the pelvic region, including prostate, uterine and urinary issues.

KILAKA MUDRA

The Sanskrit term kilaka denotes a key to a mystical secret. This mudra is particularly useful when in a puzzling situation or to maintain a harmonious relationship. Kilaka Mudra arouses a deep sense of bhakti—devotion and trust in the Infinite. The hand position signifies that while you have your own space to breathe, you are also connected to the people around you in this life as a sangha or group.

Hand Formation:

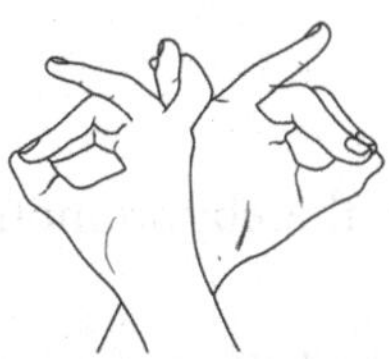

- Bring the back of both hands together in front of the chest.
- Interlock the little fingers.
- On both hands, bring the tips of the thumb, index and middle fingers together.
- Keep the ring finger straight and pointing upward at an angle.

Benefits:

- As Jala Tatva is balanced, one develops a sense of emotional security and trust, resulting in harmonious and close relationships.
- Shiva and Shakti are evoked, thus bringing about balance in relationships.
- The divinity within is evoked.

KASHYAPA MUDRA

Kashyapa Mudra, also known as Kasyapa Mudra or Tortoise Mudra, is a symbol of positivity and named after the great sage Kashyapa, who is believed to have possessed immense knowledge. The mudra should be practised for five to fifteen minutes daily for optimal benefits.

Hand Formation:

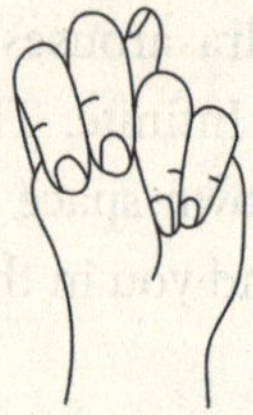

- ☞ Make a gentle fist, taking care not to curl your fingers into the palm.
- ☞ Insert the thumb between the middle and ring fingers, pressing it against the interdigital space.

Benefits:

- ☞ Protects against negative energy.
- ☞ Reduces fear, anxiety and stress.
- ☞ Enhances intuition and wisdom.
- ☞ Balances masculine and feminine energies, thereby promoting balance and harmony within.
- ☞ Activates the Mooladhara Chakra, providing a sense of grounding and stability.
- ☞ Improves focus and concentration.
- ☞ Boosts confidence and innate power.

KUNDALINI MUDRA

This is a symbol of the individual and universal self, merged together; the union of Shiva and Shakti, dormant and dynamic energy. A meditation mudra, it initiates the awakening of the dormant Kundalini energy.

Hand Formation:

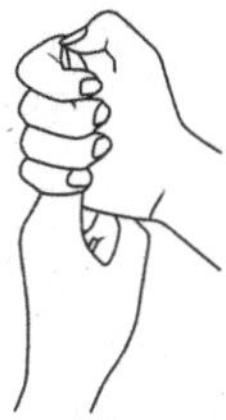

- Make a loose fist with the left hand, the thumb pressing down on the fingers.
- Stretch the left index finger upward.
- Make a fist with the right hand around the left index finger.
- Press down on top of the left index finger with the right thumb.
- Hold the hands at chest level.
- It can be practised for up to fifteen minutes, but start with two to three minutes.

Benefits:

- This mudra enhances the kundalini force, boosting overall energy levels.
- Fatigue is reduced and vitality is enhanced.
- Regular practice helps balance the endocrine system.
- Promotes reproductive and hormonal health.
- Enhances inner strength and intuition.
- It has a grounding and calming effect on the practitioner.

CHAPTER 10

Mudras for Children

Mudras energise, focus and calm the body and mind, thereby helping children regulate their emotions and feelings. Mudra practice can empower them and positively affect how they feel. They can help them improve their concentration, boost their creativity and even feel happier. These simple gestures can help children feel more balanced and in tune with their feelings.

However, mudras should be introduced to children in a playful and light environment. It should be shown to them in such a way as to spark curiosity, and you must allow them the freedom to choose what interests them. In this chapter, we will explore different hand mudras that are easy to practise and fun to learn. Children can start holding mudras from the age of five, or even younger. Showing them images of the mudras would help them understand the hand positions better.

ABHAYA MUDRA

Abhaya Mudra symbolises fearlessness, protection and peace. It is associated with safety, reassurance and the removal of obstacles.

One famous story about Lord Buddha using the Abhaya Mudra involves an encounter with a wild elephant. According to this legend, once, while Buddha was meditating in a forest, a fierce elephant, mad with rage, charged at him. The elephant's anger had been stirred, and it was on a rampage, creating chaos and fear among the people around.

Seeing the elephant charging towards him, Buddha remained calm and peaceful. Without any fear, he raised his hand in the Abhaya Mudra—the gesture for fearlessness and protection, and the wild elephant suddenly stopped in its tracks. The animal became calm and approached Buddha gently. It is said that the elephant was so moved by the Buddha's tranquil energy and compassion that it peacefully bowed down before him. There is also another interpretation that the Abhaya Mudra emits fearlessness and the elephant simply recognised that Lord Buddha did not fear it.

This story highlights the power of the Abhaya Mudra in calming negative energies and creating a sense of serenity and protection. By practising fearlessness and maintaining inner peace, even the most difficult and dangerous situations can be transformed, as shown by Buddha's use of this mudra. It teaches us that true strength comes from calmness and compassion, not force or violence.

For children, this can be very useful in difficult situations. In fact, daily practice could help them face life more courageously.

Hand Formation:

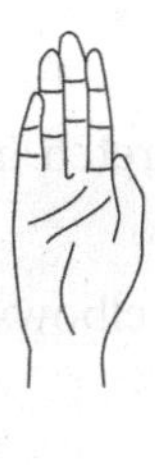

☞ Palms facing outward, raise the right hand close to the chest.
☞ Extend all the fingers.

Benefits:

- Like the name—a-bhaya (without fear)—the mudra helps you be less fearful.
- Emanates thoughts of fearlessness, influencing the people around you to develop the same attitude.
- It is a gesture of friendship; a promise of protection.

GANESHA MUDRA

Lord Ganesha is revered as the deity to be worshipped first, before any auspicious event or puja. He is believed to be both the creator and remover of obstacles—placing them in our path when necessary for our protection and clearing them when the time is right. Similarly, practising the Ganesha Mudra can invoke the same effect. One can enhance its power by taking a sankalpa (vow) or chanting a Ganesha mantra while holding the mudra. Ideally, the best time to practise this is before getting out of bed in the morning.

Hand Formation:

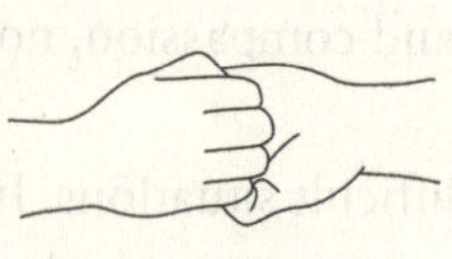

- Raise both your hands to the level of the chest, parallel to it.
- Position the left palm facing outward, away from the body, with fingers lightly folded into the palm.
- Position the right palm facing inward, towards your body, with fingers lightly folded into the palm.
- Clasp the fingers of both hands together.
- Exhale while stretching both elbows, feeling the stretch in the wrists, elbows and shoulders.
- Inhale and release the tension in the wrists, elbows, shoulders and arms.

- Repeat the inhalation and exhalation process six times.
- Switch hand positions and repeat the sequence six more times.

Benefits:

- Strengthens the fingers, hands, wrists, elbows and shoulders.
- Gives energy to the nerves and muscles.
- Increases blood circulation in the hands and shoulders.
- Common cold becomes rare; phlegm is balanced.
- Supports the strengthening of the lower body parts like the legs, knees, feet, etc.
- Activates heart muscles and lungs in the chest region; has a strong effect on the bronchial tubes.
- Boldness, activeness and the ability to mix with people is enhanced.
- As it enhances self-confidence, courage and will power, it can be very effective for students before exams and for those appearing for interviews.

PUSTAK MUDRA

Pustak Mudra is a hand gesture that is associated with knowledge, wisdom and the love of learning. The word pustak means book in Sanskrit, and this mudra is often linked with reading, writing and the pursuit of education. Pustak Mudra is connected to the brain and its neurons.

Hand Formation:

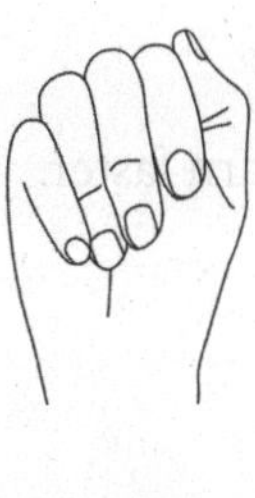

- Curl the fingers of both hands to form closed fists.
- On both hands, let the fingertips touch the mount of venus.

- Ensure that the fingernails are facing the sky.
- The thumb should touch the index finger.

Benefits:

- All the brain cells get activated, leading to an increase in concentration.
- Memory power is enhanced, making it easier for children to understand and learn concepts.
- Enhances concentration and intellectual abilities while fostering a love for learning.
- Gives them clarity and focus, and makes them feel calm.

TATVA JNANA MUDRA

As the name suggests, this mudra activates the brain cells while simultaneously permitting children to derive the benefits of the Jnana Mudra. Thus, their minds are receptive and open to scientific and philosophical thinking.

Hand Formation:

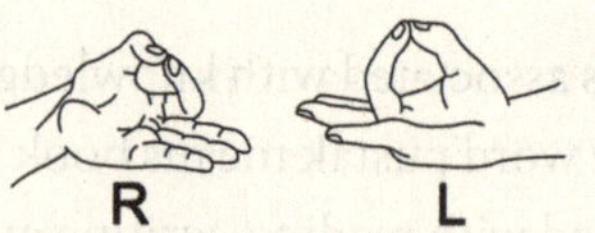

- Hold the left hand in Prithvi Mudra—the tip of the ring finger should touch the pad of the thumb.
- Form the Jnana Mudra with the right hand—the tip of the index finger should come in contact with the pad of the thumb.

Benefits:

- The mudra calms the mind, helping students learn faster.
- The brain cells are activated.

- The mind becomes open to advanced scientific thinking and complex concepts.
- Children who are physically weak benefit from Prithvi Mudra. It strengthens the human physique.

The other mudras that are highly beneficial for children include:

Hakini Mudra (Refer to Chapter 9)

Pranamam Mudra (Refer to Chapter 9)

Pankaja Mudra (Refer to Chapter 8)

CHAPTER 11

Gayatri Mudras

Enhancing Spiritual and Physical Well-Being

The human body is capable of healing itself; all we need to do is tap into that inner potential. Hand mudras are non-invasive, have no side-effects, and have a profound impact on the gross and subtle body of an individual. They help us enhance the body's healing capacity and eliminate waste and toxins. They also enhance the movement of prana shakti within the body and improve the blood flow, making one feel refreshed.

Acharya Keshav Dev, a scholar and expert in mudra science, states that in addition to the twenty-four letters of the Gayatri Mantra, Rishi Vishwamitra also devised twenty-four mudras. While they are still in use, people's ignorance has made it so that they are unable to derive benefit from them. Having conducted his own experiments, the acharya further states that performing the twenty-four Purva Mudras and eight Uttara Mudras—a total of thirty-two Gayatri Mudras—along with the Gayatri Mantra may help support overall health and well-being during cancer treatment, when combined with standard medical care.

एतां मुद्रां न जानाति, गायत्री निष्फला भवेत्।—One who does not know this mudra, the Gayatri becomes fruitless. To derive the full benefits of Gayatri Mantra, it should be chanted along with the thirty-two mudras, which leads to effective results.

The twenty-four Gayatri Mudras correspond to the twenty-four syllables in the Gayatri Mantra. According to Ayurveda, the human body is comprised of twenty-four tatvas, namely the five jnanendriyas, five karmendriyas, pancha tatvas, five tanmatras and mano-buddhi-ahankara-chitta (mind-intellect-ego-consciousness). A total of thirty-two mudras correspond to the thirty-two vertebrae on the spine. There are numerous nerves and arteries travelling through the vertebral column. When mudras are performed, these are purified.

Acharya Keshav Dev emphasises that words are not sufficient enough to express the mysterious, deep impact that Gayatri Mudras have on a person's body, mind and spirit. The Gayatri Mudras are profound practices that represent an individual's progression from the embryonic stage to nirvana. These mudras lead us through creation (dvaita or duality, involving the creator and the created) to oneness (advaita or non-duality) as illusions are dispelled. Regular practice will help the practitioner experience harmony within. Phenomenal changes can be experienced with consistent use of the Gayatri Mudras. In fact, Acharya Keshav Dev says that even if done unintentionally, one derives benefits from the use of these mudras.

NYASA

The ritual of Nyasa entails using hand mudras and touching various parts of the body, an act by which we acknowledge the presence of the divinity within. This results in bhutashuddhi (purification of the five elements) and mantra siddhi (fulfilment of the purpose of mantra chanting). Nyasa does not just heal and energise; it also bestows divine powers on the sadhaka (seeker).

Observing Nyasa before practising the twenty-four mudras helps evoke the divinity that exists inside us; it invokes a feeling of reverence. Through this, we recognise and remind ourselves every day that our body is a temple. When we practise the mudras, we connect ourselves to the divine power—even if for a short while, we push aside our daily concerns, open ourselves to receive the cosmic power, create a kavacha (shield) around us to defend against negative energies and develop visionary abilities. There are eight mudras involved in the practice of Nyasa, and each should be performed while chanting its corresponding mantra:

1. Hridaya

ॐ हृदयाय नमः (om hṛdayāya namaḥ) : The spiritual heart centre is connected to the divinity within.

Hand Formation:

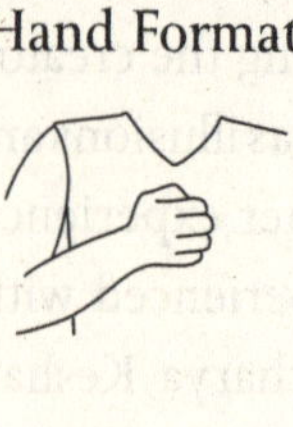

☞ Move the index finger of the right hand from the base of the thumb up to the pad of the thumb.

☞ With the fingers now in Jnana Mudra, curl the other three fingers into the palm.

☞ Bring the hand to touch the heart centre.

2. Sira

ॐ भूः शिरसे स्वाः (om bhū: śirase svāḥ): The centre of the head is associated with intuition. We offer salutations to Lord Vishnu; surrendering to the lord gives us inner security.

Hand Formation:

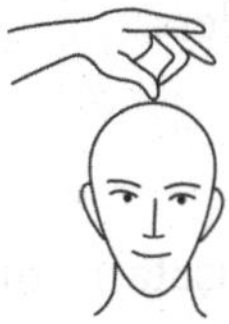

☞ On the right hand, move the pad of the thumb from the base of the index finger to its tip.

☞ One is now holding the Jnana Mudra. Keep this hand on top of the head, at the centre, with the other three fingers stretched out.

3. Shikha-Bindu

ॐ भूवः शिखायै वौषट (om bhūvaḥ śikhāyai vauṣaṭa): The seat of receiving cosmic energy; this is the spiritual gateway to anandam (bliss). In this mudra we offer salutations to Lord Rudra.

Hand Formation:

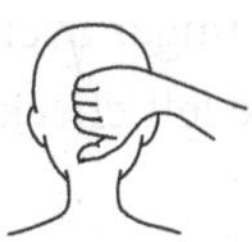

☞ On the right hand, move the pad of the thumb from the base of the middle finger to its tip.

☞ Curl all the fingers except the thumb into the palm; the thumb should remain raised.

☞ Bring the hand to the back of the head at the shikha, or bindu, with the thumb facing down.

4. Kavacha

ॐ स्वः कवचाय हुं (om svaḥ kavacāya huṃ): By creating a shield or an armour, we offer salutations to the divine light that is our armour and is protecting us.

Hand Formation:

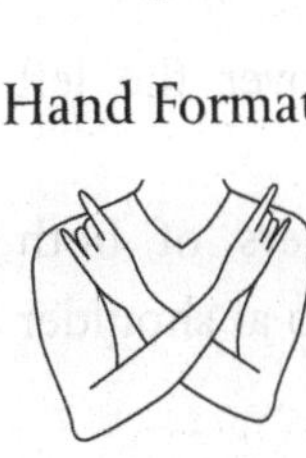

☞ On the right hand, move the pad of the thumb from the base of the ring finger to its top and hold.

- Fold in the middle and ring fingers of both hands.
- Cross both hands and place it on opposite shoulders.

5. Netratrayaaya

ॐ भूर्भुवः नेत्रत्रयाय वौषट (om bhūrbhūvaḥ netratrayāya vauṣaṭa): This mudra activates the third eye, energising and receiving blessings for divine vision. We offer salutations to the divine to protect the right and left eyes, and to open the third eye of wisdom.

Hand Formation:

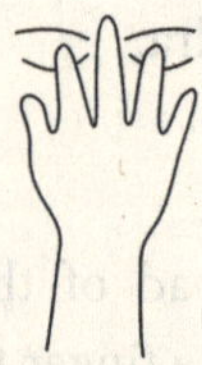

- On the right hand, move the pad of the thumb from the base of little finger to its top.
- Place the middle finger of the right hand at bhrumadhye (eyebrow centre), the index finger over the right eye, the ring finger over the left eye, the little finger on the left cheek and the thumb on the right cheek.

6. Bhurbhuvah Svah

ॐ भूर्भुवः स्वः अस्त्रायफट् (om bhūrbhūvaḥ svaḥ astrāyaphaṭ): Salutations to the all-pervading spirit to remove all evil spirits and illumine us; salutations to Mother Gayatri who is present within me; this is the weapon that burns all bondages.

Hand Formation:

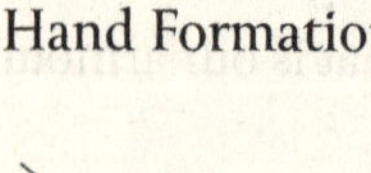

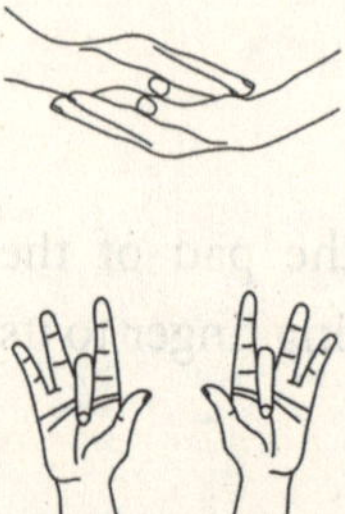

- Place the right palm over the left palm.
- Bend the middle fingers of both hands and hold them up at shoulder level.

7. Bhurbhuva Suvarom

ॐ भुर्भुवस्सुवरोम इति दिग्बन्धः (om bhurbhuvassuvaroma iti digbandhaḥ): Clapping symbolises the activation of the five elements; the sound waves produced protect the body and mind against evil thoughts and actions.

Hand Formation:

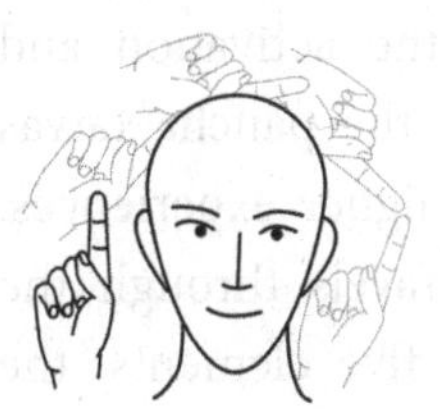

- Make a loose fist in the right hand with the thumb placed lightly over the fingers.
- Raise the index finger.
- Move it around the head in a clockwise direction.
- Clap the palm of the left hand with the right index and middle fingers.

One is now able to invoke Vedmatha Gayatri within; she is the source of all creation, the embodiment of all wisdom. 'May my mind meditate on you, Vedmatha', and with these words we establish Vedmatha Gayatri in our heart.

By holding these mudras, one attains calmness and is prepared for the Purva Mudras, the chanting of the Gayatri Mantra and finally, to hold the Uttara Mudras.

PURVA MUDRAS

The twenty-four Purva Mudras represent the journey of a human from the embryo to the unfolding of the consciousness, and finally, enlightenment. These mudras symbolise the four stages of human life:

Birth: when physical needs are important and sought out.

Brahmacharya: where the process of acquiring knowledge occurs; the journey from darkness to light.

Jnana marga: where one lives a disciplined life, getting involved in deeper studies and the gaining of Vedic knowledge.

Self-realisation: when you merge with the Parabrahman, the consciousness.

The first seventeen mudras focus on the activation and energising of the nadis and chakras. Once the pancha tatvas are balanced, the practitioner is ready for higher experiences. Through these twenty-four mudras, one travels through the process of evolution, the balancing of the five elements, the activation of the subtle body, and ultimately, merges with the Absolute. The names of the twenty-four Purva Mudras should be chanted while holding the mudras themselves:

सुमुखं सम्पुटं चैव विततं विस्तृतं तथा
द्विमुखं त्रिमुखं चैव चतुः पंच मुखं तथा
षण्मुख अधोमुखं चैव व्यापकांजलिकं तथा
शकटं यमपाशंच ग्रन्थितं चोन्मुखोन्मुखं
प्रलंबं मुष्ठिकं चैव मत्स्यः कूर्मो वराहकम्सिं
हाक्रांतं महाक्रांतं मुद्गरं पल्लवं तथा

sumukhaṃ sampuṭaṃ caiva vitataṃ vistṛtaṃ tathā
dvimukhaṃ trimukhaṃ caiva catuḥ paṃca mukhaṃ tathā
ṣaṇmukha adhomukhaṃ caiva vyāpakāṃjalikaṃ tathā
śakaṭaṃ yamapāśaṃca granthitaṃ conmukhonmukhaṃ
pralaṃbaṃ muṣṭhikaṃ caiva matsyaḥ kūrmo varāhakam
siṃhākrāṃtaṃ mahākrāṃtaṃ mudgaraṃ pallavaṃ tathā

SUMUKHAM MUDRA

This mudra represents the bindu—the oneness or wholeness of the universe before it manifested as what it is today. This marks the start of evolution. Sumukham Mudra symbolises the iccha (intention) and the energy to create, and prepares the body and mind for meditation, enhancing focus and energy flow.

Hand Formation:

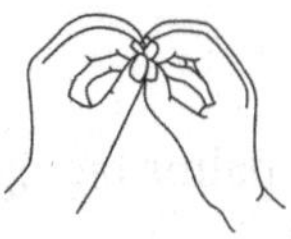

- Hold the Samana Mudra with both hands.
- Bring both the hands together, letting the fingertips touch.

SAMPUTAM MUDRA

This mudra symbolises the stage of expansion. Once the iccha has been identified, the bindu expands into a bud—a storehouse of knowledge. The elongated fingers signify the knowledge within every individual. At the physical level, Samputam Mudra helps in attaining mental clarity and stability. This a prayer to invoke the merging of the knowledge within oneself with the Absolute.

Hand Formation:

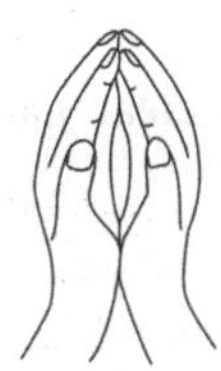

- Bring both the hands together, with each fingertip—except the thumbs—touching its counterpart on the opposite hand.
- The thumbs should stay parallel to each other.
- The fingers should be close together and slightly curved such that a hollow is created between the palms.

VITATAM MUDRA

The fingers are open in this mudra, demonstrating the gradual opening up of the bud when iccha shakti is converted into kriya shakti. The intention to create is now progressing towards action. At this stage, indriyas and gross elements become visible. At the physical level, this mudra aids in emotional release and the resulting growth that comes with clarity of feelings.

Hand Formation:

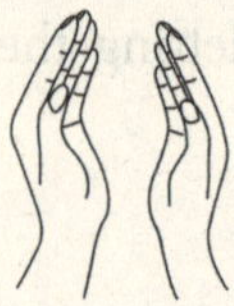

☞ Keep both hands slightly apart, palms facing each other—signifying the bud opening up.

☞ The fingers should remain slightly cupped.

VISTRUTAM MUDRA

Further expansion of the universe takes place, and the positioning of the hands symbolises the universe. The bud is now ready to bloom—to expand its awareness and consciousness. This mudra symbolises the connection of the individual to the universe.

Hand Formation:

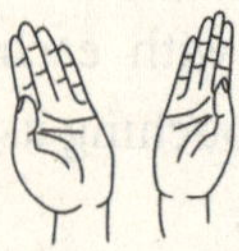

☞ Both hands are parted, leaving a clear gap between them.

The four mudras above represent the evolutionary stages in human life.

DVIMUKHAM MUDRA

This mudra symbolises the duality: Purusha—the formless and that without attributes; and Prakriti—with many forms and attributes. Thus, this mudra balances the duality within and promotes harmony between thoughts and emotions.

Hand Formation:

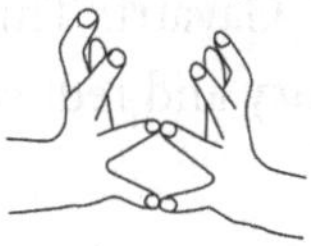

- Bring the ring and little fingers of both hands in touch with each other.
- The other fingers remain free and apart from each other.

TRIMUKHAM MUDRA

This mudra represents the combined energy of the Trinity—Brahma, Vishnu and Shiva. It is the combined energy of iccha shakti, jnana shakti and kriya shakti; it enhances communication as middle fingers—representing Akasha Tatva and hence, responsible for verbal communication—now touch each other.

Hand Formation:

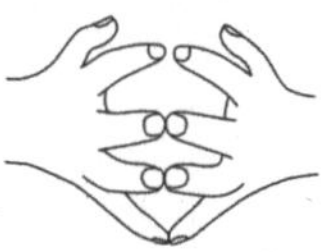

- Hold the Dvimukham Mudra.
- Bring the middle fingers of both hands in contact with each other.

CHATURMUKHAM MUDRA

This mudra represents the four Vedas and the four purusharthas—dharma, artha, kama and moksha. At the physical level, it helps release emotions and attain mental stability.

Hand Formation:

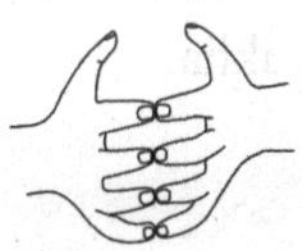

- Hold the Trimukham Mudra.
- Bring the index fingers of both hands in contact with each other.

PANCHAMUKHAM MUDRA

All the five fingers are joined together, symbolising the pancha tatvas, the pancha pranas and the five faces of Gayatri. This mudra helps stimulate the senses, revitalise memory and reduce fatigue.

Hand Formation:

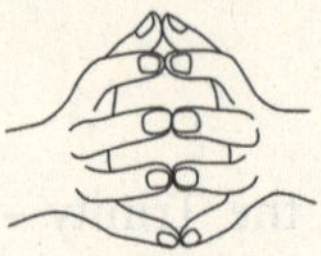

- Hold the Chaturmukham Mudra.
- Bring the thumbs of both hands in contact with each other.

The mudras from Dvimukham to Panchamukham aid in the release of anger and frustration, thereby leading to the attainment of brahmacharya. One becomes capable of releasing their emotions once the process of acquiring knowledge has begun; it is a part of the journey from darkness to light.

SHANMUKHAM MUDRA

Shanmukha is another name for Lord Kartikeya, who was born after great tapas. Hence, this mudra represents great tapas, activating the six energy centres within the body. Shanmukham Mudra invokes the senses and improves perception.

Hand Formation:

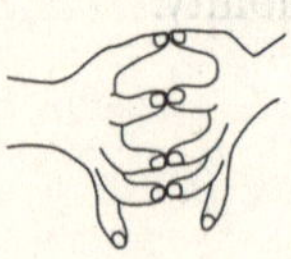

- Hold the Panchamukham Mudra.
- Release the contact between the little fingers and stretch them downward—this depicts the six faces of Shanmukha.

ADHOMUKHAM MUDRA

The mind by its nature is in constant motion. In this mudra, the fingers point downward, representing the process of being sucked into the material world as we are pulled into creation. At the physical level, this mudra encourages self-reflection.

Hand Formation:

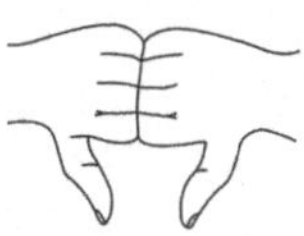

☞ Bring the knuckles of both hands, except the thumbs, into contact.

☞ Point all the fingers, including the thumb, downward.

VYAPAKANJALIKAM MUDRA

The word vyapaka means expansion. The process of evolution begins here. This mudra enhances energy flow throughout the body.

Hand Formation:

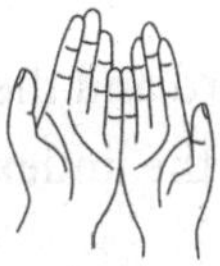

☞ Bring both palms together, open and facing upward, with the sides touching.

SAKATAM MUDRA

The body is a vehicle for the atma (soul) and represents the beginning of the journey with the trigunas (the three attributes of nature). The three folded fingers represent the trigunas, which need to be overcome so as to reach a state of anandam; one must attain the status of trigunatheetham (beyond the three attributes). At the physical level, this mudra promotes digestion and the metabolic process.

Hand Formation:

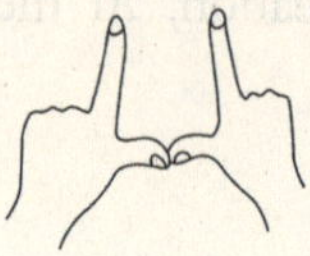

- Position the hands with the palms facing downward.
- Bring the tips of both thumbs in contact with each other.
- Extend the index fingers.
- Curl the remaining fingers into the palm.

YAMAPASHAM MUDRA

This mudra signifies the release of pasham (bondage)—release from the janana-marana cycle (cycle of birth and death). This requires control over our desires, which can be achieved through focus and discipline. The practice of this mudra can help release the pasham that binds us.

Hand Formation:

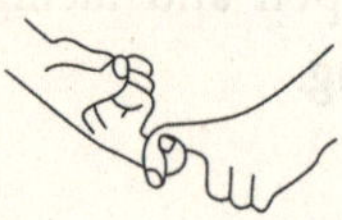

- With the left palm facing downward and the right palm facing upward, lock the index fingers of both hands together.
- Loosely fold the other fingers into the palm.

GRANTHITAM MUDRA

The fingers clasped together assist in releasing the tension and blockages in the body. This mudra symbolises the assimilation of strength and the power to transcend the mind and grow beyond it.

Hand Formation:

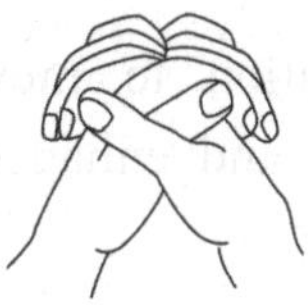

☞ Thread the fingers of both hands between each other so that the hands are clasped and form a closed fist.

CHONMUKHONMUKHAM MUDRA

This mudra symbolises that one should remain open to new experiences and perspectives in life. Adaptability is a quality that encourages one to accept and move towards the unknown and unseen.

Hand Formation:

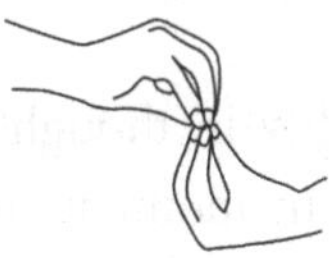

☞ Form the Samana Mudra with both hands.

☞ Place the right hand over the left while holding this mudra, the fingertips of both hands touching each other.

☞ Immediately reverse the hand positions so that the left hand is over the right.

PRALAMBAM MUDRA

This mudra symbolises expanding the consciousness and growing beyond. This can be achieved by enhancing energy levels and vitality, which is what the mudra leads one to.

Hand Formation:

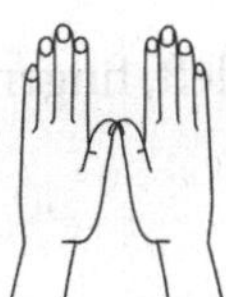

☞ Hold both hands with the palms facing downward.

☞ Bring the thumbs of both hands into contact with each other.

MUSHTIKAM MUDRA

Mushtikam represents resolve, the determination to move forward; it grants strength, boosts confidence and enhances willpower.

Hand Formation:

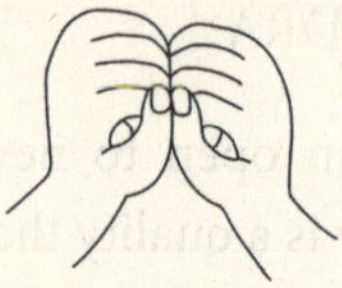

☞ Fold the fingers of both hands into the palms.

☞ Bring the folded fingers into contact with each other by the middle joints of the fingers.

☞ Keep the thumbs straight and parallel to each other.

MATSYAM MUDRA

The water element is activated, enhancing fluidity in thoughts and actions. This enables one to be adaptable. In moments of doubt, this mudra helps one swim across the bhavasaagara (ocean of life) fearlessly, without being affected by the consequences. This also represents the first of the dasavatara of Maha Vishnu. A fish lives in the water without becoming entangled in the mud beneath. At the physical level, his mudra helps us get rid of the six negativities—kama (lust), krodha (anger), lobha (greed), moha (delusion), mada (pride) and matsarya (jealousy).

Hand Formation:

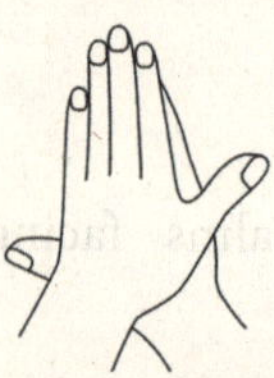

☞ Keep both palms facing downward, parallel to the floor.

☞ Rest the right palm on top of the left, fingers held close together.

☞ Extend the thumbs out to the sides.

KURMAM MUDRA

Kurmam, a tortoise, is comfortable both on land and in water, representing the adaptability invoked by this mudra. Kurmam is also known for withdrawing into itself—pratyahara—which is protection against negative energies. This mudra also helps us develop patience. Moreover, a tortoise takes fewer number of breaths than most other living creatures on Earth. It thus encourages us to engage in pranayama so that our respiration rate is reduced.

Hand Formation:

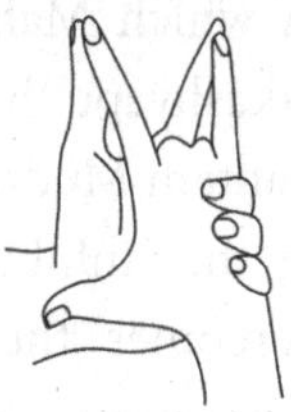

- ☞ Left hand: palm facing upward, keep the thumb and index finger straight.
- ☞ Right hand: palm facing downward, fold the middle and ring fingers into it.
- ☞ Rest the right thumb at the base of the left wrist, parallel to the length of the arm.
- ☞ Touch the right index finger to the left thumb.
- ☞ Rest the right little finger on the left index finger.
- ☞ Curl the middle, ring and little fingers of the left hand over the back of the right.

VARAHAKAM MUDRA

Varaha, another Vishnu avatara, saved humanity by lifting the Earth from the cosmic ocean. This mudra enhances stability in life and helps keep you grounded.

Hand Formation:

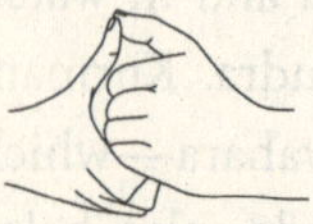

- Keep the right palm facing upward and the left facing downward.
- Fold the four fingers of the right hand into the palm.
- Fold the four fingers of the left hand over and around the four fingers of the right.
- Bring the pads of the two thumbs into contact with each other.

SIMHAKRANTAM MUDRA

This mudra indicates the Narasimha avatara, in which Maha Vishnu clawed away the six negativities of Hiranyakashyapu that were destroying human beings. With the Simhakrantam Mudra, the forces of ego and arrogance—and anything that inhibits spiritual progress—are destroyed, and one overcomes their fears. According to Acharya Keshav Dev, one becomes brave and mighty like a lion.

Hand Formation:

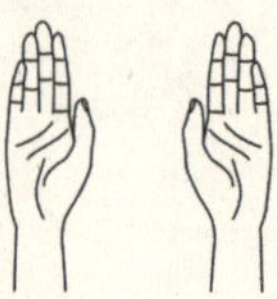

- Place both hands on either side of the face with the palms tilted slightly towards it and with fingers bent slightly, like a lion's claw.

MAHAKRANTAM MUDRA

Representing transformation and change, this mudra offers protection, as the jeeva (jivatma) is now free from egoistic tendencies. It removes ignorance and prepares one for the spiritual journey.

Hand Formation:

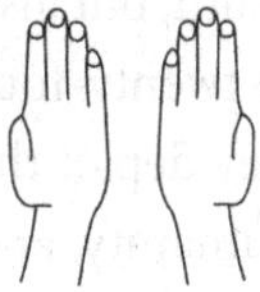

☞ Place both hands on either side of your face, palms facing the ears, at a distance of six to seven inches.

MUDGARAM MUDRA

This mudra indicates the gadaa—the mace, Lord Hanuman's weapon. It represents the shakti flowing through the upright spine, encouraging the development of morals and spiritual values. It gives you clarity of thought and stability in life.

Hand Formation:

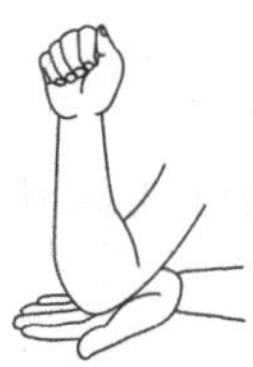

☞ Form a fist with the right hand (representing the base of the skull).

☞ Keep the upper right arm upright (symbolising a straight spine).

☞ Cup the palm of the left hand and place it under the right elbow.

PALLAVAM MUDRA

This mudra symbolises the blossoming of the Sahasrara Chakra, similar to how a bud expands and grows spiritually.

Hand Formation:

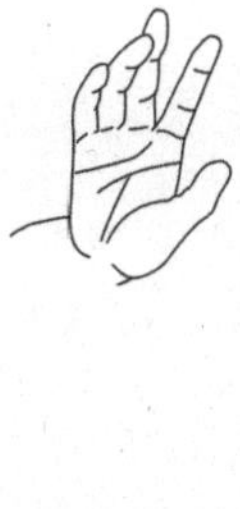

☞ Cup the right hand and hold it facing outward.

☞ Keep the hand at chest level.

When practised regularly alongside the chanting of the Gayatri Mantra, these mudras not only facilitate physical health, but also support mental clarity and emotional balance. The twenty-four Purva Mudras reveal ancient Vedic knowledge—they depict the evolution of the consciousness from animality to humanity, and ultimately to divinity. People travel from dvaitam (duality) to advaitam (non-dualism).

After the Purva Mudras, the Gayatri Mantra is to be chanted ten times:

ॐ भूर्भुवः स्वः तत्सवितुर्वरेण्यं
भर्गो देवस्य धीमही धियो योनः प्रचोदयात् ।

om bhūrbhuvaḥ svaḥ tatsaviturvareṇyam
bhargo devasya dhīmahī dhiyo yonaḥ pracodayāt |

UTTARA MUDRAS

As the Uttara Mudras are held, the following mantra should be chanted:

सुरभी ज्ञान वैराग्यं योनि शंखोत पंकजं
लिंगं निर्वाणकं चैव जपांतेष्टौ प्रदर्शयेत्
ॐ शान्तिः शान्तिः शान्तिः

surabhī jñāna vairāgyaṃ yoni śaṃkhota paṃkajaṃ
liṃgaṃ nirvāṇakaṃ caiva japāṃteṣṭau pradarśayet
oṁ śāntiḥ śāntiḥ śāntiḥ

SURABHI MUDRA

For a detailed explanation of this mudra, refer to Chapter 8.

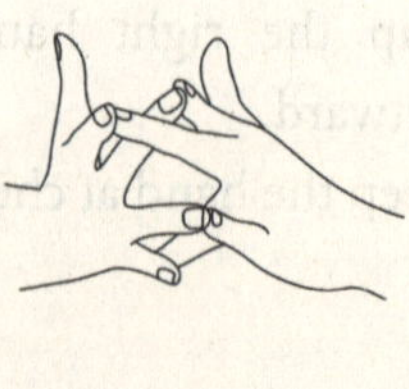

JNANA MUDRA

For a detailed explanation of this mudra, refer to Chapter 7.

Hand formation:

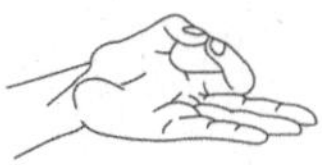

- Place the right hand in Jnana Mudra at the heart centre.
- Place the left hand in Jnana Mudra and rest it on the left knee.

VAIRAGYA MUDRA

Hand Formation:

- Place both hands in Jnana Mudra and rest them on the knees.

YONI MUDRA

For a detailed explanation of this mudra, refer to Chapter 8.

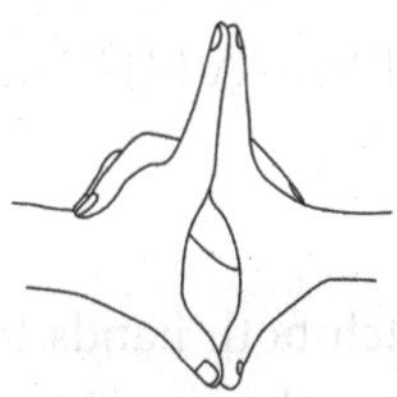

SHANKHA MUDRA

For a detailed explanation of this mudra, refer to Chapter 8.

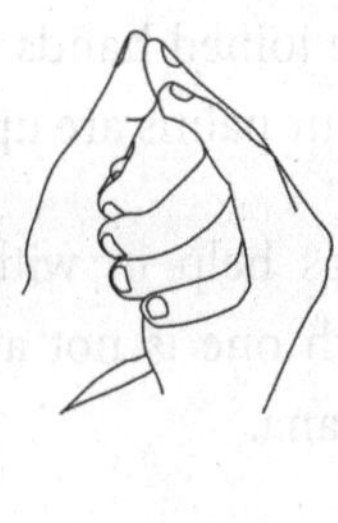

PANKAJA MUDRA

For a detailed explanation of this mudra, refer to Chapter 8.

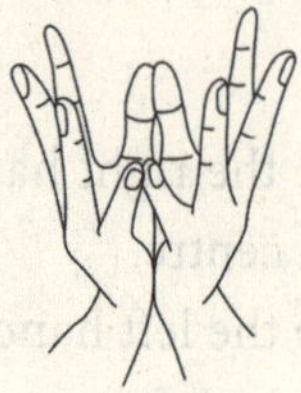

LINGA MUDRA

For a detailed explanation of this mudra, refer to Chapter 8.

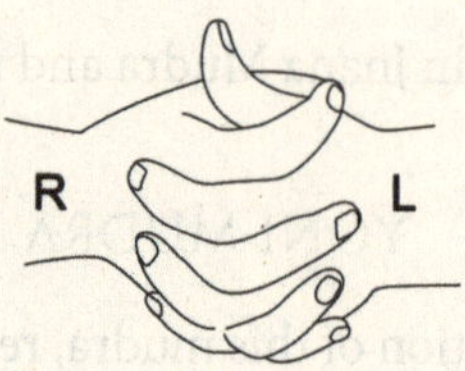

NIRVANA MUDRA

Hand Formation:

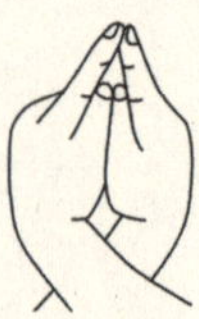

- ☞ Stretch both hands forward with the backs of the palms touching.
- ☞ Bring the right palm over the left so that the hands cross at the wrists and both palms come into contact.
- ☞ While keeping both palms together, rotate the forearms at the elbows, swinging the joined hands downward in an arc and then upward until your palms are upright.

The eight Uttara Mudras help in withdrawing all the senses, attaining a state in which one is not affected by delusions and desires, and reaches nirvana.

The jivatma journeys with the desire to attain happiness (Surabhi Mudra), and through jnanam (Jnana Mudra), one attains vairagya (Vairagya Mudra). One is then able to withdraw within (Yoni Mudra) and be free from the janana-marana cycle. The truth—the naada brahmam—OM (Shankha Mudra) then blossoms like a Pankaja Satchitananda (Pankaja Mudra) and attains the status of Lingam—formless, the symbol of Lord Shiva—(Linga Mudra), and then finally achieves niravana—the very purpose of human life (Nirvana Mudra).

A query that often arises is whether these mudras can support individuals suffering from cancer and undergoing treatment.

Mudras are not a substitute for conventional cancer treatment. But when practised alongside prescribed cancer care, some individuals have reported benefits such as improved health, reduced anxiety, clarity of mind, etc. The following mudras are particularly recommended for those undergoing treatments like radiation or chemotherapy:

Samana Mudra: this mudra is reported to help make the body receptive to treatment.

Prana Mudra: users report that this mudra can aid in alleviating lethargy and mental fatigue.

It is suggested that practising the two mudras for fifteen minutes, thrice a day, will bring you benefits.

CHAPTER 12

The Synergy of Mudras, Visualisation and Affirmations

Mudras, or sacred hand gestures, have been integral to spiritual and healing practices in various traditions, especially in yoga and Ayurveda. By combining mudras with visualisation and affirmations, we can enhance their power and create a holistic tool for transforming the mind, body and energy systems. In this chapter we explore this synergy by focusing on Surabhi Mudra and Kubera Mudra, along with the processes of visualisation and affirmations.

MUDRAS AND VISUALISATION

Mudras are independent yoganga that activate specific energy channels in the body, helping to restore balance and enhance a person's physical, mental and spiritual well-being. Each mudra directs the flow of energy in a unique way. Only after the mind is balanced can visualisation work.

CREATING AN INTENTION

However, before visualisation, one must understand how to set the right intention. We can shape our life the way we want—we can shape our experiences, our relationships and our successes. However, this requires both an unshakeable faith in oneself and the determination to succeed.

Creating an intention requires desire, belief and acceptance. One must be practical and avoid pursuing unrealistic desires.

You may not find success initially. Our mind is accustomed to negative images and thought patterns. Once we get rid of these, we learn to create the right intention.

VISUALISATION: A TOOL FOR MANIFESTATION

When the mind is steady, it can create the right intention. Visualisation is a powerful technique that harnesses the imagination to create mental images capable of influencing our reality. While visualisation is not easy, according to Rajendar Menen (2016), 'sustained and honest practice' can help achieve results (p. 25). The power of the mind and that of visual imagery has been spoken of in Vedic scriptures. In yogic and meditative practices, it is used to strengthen the connection between mind and energy, allowing us to focus our intent and shape our outcomes.

Ancient texts like the *Yoga Sutras of Patanjali* emphasise the power of mental concentration and visualisation as tools to attain samadhi (spiritual realisation). Rishi Patanjali speaks about the practice of dharana (concentration) and dhyana (meditation), which are closely related to visualisation. The act of focusing through images or mantras is said to purify the mind and lead to higher states of consciousness.

For instance, *Patanjali Yoga Sutra* (3.2) state: *Tatra pratyaya-eka-tanata dhyanam* [Meditation (dhyanam) is the uninterrupted flow of the mind towards that object]. Verses like these imply that visualisation helps develop one-pointed concentration and leads one to a higher state of consciousness. Thus, apart from achieving goals such as physical and mental well-being, and acquiring material possessions, visualisation helps in harnessing the brain's full potential.

Swami Paramahansa Yogananda (1998) speaks about the importance of visualisation in spiritual practices, particularly to align oneself with the divine energies. He emphasises that focusing the mind with clear intention can help transform inner reality, and consequently lead to outer changes.

Gertrud Hirschi (2016) states, 'If we can clearly express what we do not want and definitively formulate our wishes and needs, this can already be the beginning of a new order in life' (p. 25). Mudras influence the brain waves, so when a wish-fulfilling mudra is held with full concentration, the power of imagination is enhanced and one works in alignment with the wishes.

AFFIRMATIONS: REWIRING THE MIND

Affirmations are short, positive statements that we repeat consciously to reshape our thought patterns. According to Vedantic philosophy and modern psychology, the mind is malleable, and repetitive positive thoughts can reprogramme the subconscious. Affirmations work like mantras, helping to purify our negative mindset and reinforce new, empowering beliefs. They help remove the pessimistic thought patterns and impressions present in the inner mind.

Using affirmations alongside visualisation works wonders. Repeat your affirmations while visualising, ideally one to three times daily—or simply whenever you find time during the day. Start with small things first before proceeding to larger things. Voice your affirmations out loud. Affirmations should be made with conviction, dedication and the utmost faith.

This practice is beneficial for most people; students, people with a particular focus (career, marriage, etc.)—anybody with a goal.

* * *

There are two mudras that support the fulfilment of wishes and needs: Surabhi Mudra and Kubera Mudra.

SURABHI MUDRA: THE WISH-FULFILLING GESTURE

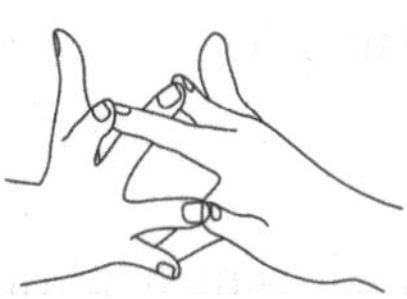

Surabhi Mudra (refer to Chapter 8), also known as the Kamadhenu Mudra (named after the wish-fulfilling cow in Hindu mythology), is one of the most powerful mudras for balancing the five elements in the body. It is especially beneficial for reducing stress, and improving the health of the respiratory system and digestive tract. It is believed to bring material and spiritual abundance. At the spiritual level, this means that one has transcended all desires and attained contentment; there are no further desires to be fulfilled.

Visualisation with Surabhi Mudra:

By combining the power of Surabhi Mudra, a clear visualisation and a positive affirmation, you magnify the energy of manifestation, creating a space for abundance to enter your life.

A woman who attended my intensive hand mudra course in May 2024 shared this mudra with her daughter, who was seeking career progression in the UK. She practised the Surabhi Mudra with visualisation and affirmation while trying to secure a band 6 role as a prison officer—a difficult task, especially considering her band 4 position. Just two days after the interview, she received news that she had been selected!

Another woman in the UK, a yoga teacher, has told me of her small successes. She used the technique for everyday things, like getting household items at her preferred price and similar situations. Small success gives one the confidence to use the technique for higher gains.

Surabhi Mudra, combined with visualisation and affirmations, can be applied for both oneself and for others—for healing physical and mental ailments, as well as for achieving material and spiritual gains. It is based on the principle, यथा चिन्ता तथा स्थिति: (yathā cintā tathā sthiti:)—as one thinks, so one becomes. This is a concept deeply rooted in the Upanishadic principles.

Affirmation with Surabhi Mudra

☞ Create an intention. Write it as a short, clear sentence with no ambiguities. The intention should be clearly stated on the first day and doesn't need to be repeated daily. After the first day, keep the written note somewhere safe.

☞ Intentions are always in the past or present, even though the meaning might be future oriented. For example, 'I see my solar panel business firmly established by the end of November 2026', not 'I will start my own business next year.'

☞ Hold the Surabhi Mudra and visualise the events as you wish them to unfold. Let the mind take you wherever it wants to travel. Ideally, remain in this state for at least fifteen minutes but do not stop if the mind continues to visualise.

- Repeat the affirmation.
- Do this for twenty-one days before stopping.

KUBERA MUDRA: THE MUDRA OF MANIFESTATION

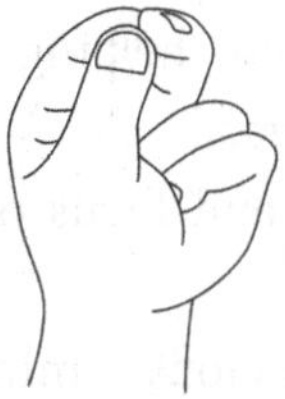

Named after Kubera, the god of wealth in Hindu mythology, Kubera Mudra (refer to Chapter 8) is a potent gesture for manifesting desires and intentions. It is particularly useful for focusing energy on specific goals, irrespective of whether they are material, emotional or spiritual. It helps generate positive thoughts and thus, is effective in sorting out dilemmas, improving discriminatory powers and, true to its name, in attracting wealth.

Kubera Mudra gives you the courage to make projects succeed. Since the energy is concentrated, one can direct it wherever one wants. It strengthens resolve and provides you with the confidence and calm necessary to proceed.

Visualisation with Kubera Mudra:

Visualise yourself already in possession of what you are trying to manifest. For instance, if you are manifesting financial abundance, imagine yourself surrounded by wealth, prosperity and opportunities. Focus on feeling the emotions of fulfilment and gratitude.

Affirmation for Kubera Mudra:

'I attract wealth easily, and money flows to me from both expected and unexpected sources.'

By performing the Kubera Mudra with intention and affirming your goals, you create a powerful synergy that accelerates the manifestation process.

THE SYNERGY: HOW MUDRAS, VISUALISATION AND AFFIRMATIONS WORK TOGETHER

When used in combination, mudras, visualisation and affirmations create a multi-layered system for self-transformation. Each of these elements works on different aspects of our being:

- Mudras influence the body's energy channels, helping to balance the physical, mental and spiritual layers.
- Visualisation helps us direct mental energy and focus our intent on the desired outcome.
- Affirmations reprogramme the subconscious mind, reinforcing positive mental patterns and freeing us from limiting beliefs.

The Yoga Sutras of Patanjali describe the importance of mental clarity and focus (dharana) in achieving spiritual growth. Visualisation aids in this by concentrating our mental energies, while affirmations work to rewrite negative programming, aligning our thoughts with our deepest desires. When these practices are combined with mudras, they activate the subtle energy channels in the body, enhancing the impact of both.

KEY TEXTS ON VISUALISATION AND AFFIRMATIONS

- The Vedas and the Upanishads: These ancient texts contain references to mantras and the power of sound, and refers to them as a force that shapes reality. Affirmations are a form of modern-day mantra, using the same principles of invoking change through words.
- *The Power of Now* by Eckhart Tolle: While not directly focused on visualisation or affirmations, Tolle's teachings about living in the present moment emphasise how cultivating mindful awareness and intention can transform our perception and unlock new possibilities.

- *The Secret* by Rhonda Byrne: This book popularised the concept of the 'Law of Attraction', which is the idea that by focusing on positive thoughts and visualising desired outcomes, you can attract those things into your life. It includes insights into how visualisation and affirmations can manifest your desires.
- *You Can Heal Your Life* by Louise Hay: Louise Hay's book is an essential read for anyone interested in affirmations and self-healing. She explains how thoughts and beliefs shape your reality, and offers powerful affirmations that can be used to overcome negative thought patterns and heal physical ailments.
- *Creative Visualisation* by Shakti Gawain: This book is dedicated to the power of visualisation and how it can be used for personal growth, success and healing. It provides techniques and exercises that teach you how to use visualisation to achieve your goals and create a better life.

LAW OF ATTRACTION AND HOW IT WORKS

1. You are the most powerful magnet on earth and you can direct your prana to wherever your awareness is; your energy goes where your focus is. The magnetic energy is emitted through your thoughts. You become what you think, so hold on to the thoughts about what you want or what you want to be, and make them your most dominant thoughts.
2. The principal reasons why people do not achieve what they manifest is a lack of confidence and excessive effort. It is also because we do not know how the subconscious mind works. We always think of what we do not want, rather than what we do want—and this is precisely why the Law of Attraction brings us what we do not want. Be sure about what you do not

want, then focus all your energy and attention on what you do want in your life.

3. As we have learnt through meditation, energy follows where your attention goes. We have the power to direct energy wherever we choose. When negative thoughts arise, flip them into their positive counterparts. Never tell yourself that you cannot do something; instead, affirm, 'Yes, I can.'
4. Words and thoughts are incredibly powerful tools—use them wisely to manifest the life you desire. Stop repeatedly focusing on your problems and negative circumstances, as doing so only strengthens them—both for you and for those who hear you.
5. Replace negative language with empowering words that reflect your aspirations. For example, if you find yourself saying, 'I am overweight', reframe it to, 'I am gradually losing weight and will soon reach my ideal weight.' Consistently remind yourself of who you want to be and visualise the person you aim to become.
6. Speak from the heart and avoid using hurtful words, as they often stem from fear. Reflect on the words you choose: will they help or hinder your growth? What you say floats out into the universe and returns to you multiplied. Every word you speak first manifests on the mental plane before becoming reality on the physical plane.
7. Visualisation involves using the power of thought to create mental images that design your future. To begin manifesting, recognise the distinction between awareness and the mind. We are not our minds; we are the awareness that moves through them. Once you understand this, you can direct your awareness wherever you choose. Where your awareness goes, energy flows—and with it, you can influence the flow of your energy.

8. Energy is like water; it grows whatever you direct it at. If you focus your energy on positive things, they will grow. If you focus on negativity, that will expand as well. When your awareness is fixed on your goals, energy flows into them, and you start seeing manifestations in your life.
9. Be mindful and intentional about where you spend your energy. You only have a limited amount of energy each day, so assess your life and decide how to allocate it wisely among the people and things that matter most to you. What you manifest in your life is directly related to where and how much energy you invest.

By combining Surabhi Mudra, Kubera Mudra, visualisation techniques and positive affirmations, we can align our physical and energetic bodies with our goals. This practice harmonises the mind, body and soul, creating an ideal environment for manifesting both material and spiritual abundance. As ancient teachings and modern psychology show, our thoughts, emotions and actions are deeply intertwined, and by consciously working with them, we can create profound shifts in our lives.

Incorporating these practices into your daily routine is a simple yet powerful way to enhance your overall well-being, focus your energy and bring your deepest intentions to life.

Appendix

Index of Mudras

These are the mudra practices that, in the author's experience, were found to be helpful for the specified concerns.

Concern	Mudras
Acne/Blackheads	Prithvi Mudra + Jala Mudra. Hold hands in Samana Mudra and place it on acne for 15 minutes
Acidity	Surabhi Mudra/Apana Vayu Mudra + Prana Mudra
Allergy	Jala Mudra + Shankha Mudra/Bhramara Mudra
Alzheimer's	Jnana Mudra (15 min) + Vyana Mudra (15 min) + Prana Mudra (15 min)
Anemia	Prithvi Mudra + Prana Mudra
Anxiety	Bhairava Mudra + Jnana Mudra + Prana Mudra
Arthritis	Keela Mudra + Vayu Mudra + Prana Mudra
Asthma	Linga Mudra + Pooshana Mudra OR Asthma Mudra
Auto Immune System	Mukula Mudra
Bile Issues	Surabhi Mudra + Prana Mudra
Boils	Jala Mudra + Prana Mudra
Blood Circulation	Vyana Mudra + Prana Mudra
Blood Impurity	Prithvi Mudra

Concern	Mudras
Blood Pressure	Kanishta Mudra
Cancer Care	Gayatri Mudras – set of 32 (can be taught separately)
Cataract	Surya Mudra + Prana Mudra
Cervical Spondylitis	Ganesha Mudra + Vayu Mudra + Prana Mudra + Hold Samana Mudra on the area for 15 min
Cerebral Palsy	Vayu Mudra + Prana Mudra + Jnana Mudra
Chest Pain	Apana Vayu Mudra + Akasha Mudra
Cholesterol	Surya Mudra + Prana Mudra
Cold	Linga Mudra + Surya Mudra
Concentration	Bhairava Mudra + Jnana Mudra
Congestion (Chest)	Linga Mudra + Prana Mudra
Constipation	Suchi Mudra/Apana Mudra + Apana Vayu Mudra
Corns	Surya Mudra + Place Samana Mudra over the corn
Cough (dry)	Jala Mudra
Cough (wet)	Linga Mudra + Surya Mudra
Cracked (dry) Skin	Jala Mudra + Prithvi Mudra
Cramps/Muscle Catch	Jala Mudra + Prana Mudra
Cyst in the Uterus	Jalodhara Nashaka Mudra + Uttara Bodhi Mudra + Prana Mudra
Dehydration	Jala Vardhaka Mudra
Depression	Bhairava Mudra + Jnana Mudra + Prana Mudra
Diabetes	Apana Mudra + Prana Mudra
Diarrhoea	Jalodhara Nashaka Mudra + Apana Mudra
Digestion	Maatangi Mudra + Apana Mudra/Apana Mudra + Pooshana Mudra + Surya Mudra
Dilemma in Selection	Kubera Mudra
Ear Problems	Shoonya Mudra + Akasha Mudra
Eczema/Skin Issues	Jala Mudra + Prana Mudra
Energy	Jnana Mudra + Prithvi Mudra + Prana Mudra
Endometriosis/PCOD	Sahaja Shankha Mudra (at the navel) + Shankha Mudra (both mudras with both hands)

Concern	Mudras
Epilepsy	Mrigi Mudra + Jnana Mudra + Prana Mudra
Excess Sweating	Apana Vayu Mudra + Vyana Mudra
Eyes	Surya Mudra + Samana Mudra
Eye Redness	Prana Mudra
Fibroid	Yoni Mudra + Linga Mudra
Fearlessness	Abhaya Mudra
Fever + Cold	Surya Mudra + Pankaja Mudra
Fungal Infection	Fungus Mudra ((5 min + 8 min + 12 min) x 3)
Gastroenteritis	Jala Mudra
Gall Bladder Pain/Stone	Pooshana Mudra + Hold Samana Mudra on the region for 15 min
Glaucoma	Jnana Mudra + Prana Mudra + Hold Samana Mudra on the eyes for 15 min
Gout	Surabhi Mudra + Vayu Mudra + Prana Mudra
Gynecological Issues	Uttara Bodhi Mudra + Shoonya Vayu Mudra
Hair Greying (untimely)/ Hair Fall	Prithvi Mudra (50 min) + Prana Mudra
Heart Problems	Akasha Mudra (15 min) + Apana Vayu Mudra (15 min) + Prana Mudra (15 min)
Heart Attack	Apana Vayu Mudra (50 min) + Prana Mudra
Hernia	Vayu Mudra + Prithvi Mudra + Prana Mudra
Hemoglobin	Jala Mudra + Garuda Mudra + Prana Mudra
Herpes	Herpes Mudra
Hiccups	Apana Vayu Mudra
Hormonal Imbalance	Ushas Mudra
Hyperacidity	Surabhi Mudra + Apana Vayu Mudra + Prithvi Mudra
IBS	Shoonya Vayu Mudra + Prithvi Mudra
Illness Prevention	Shoonya Vayu Mudra
Immunity	Pooshana Mudra + Prana Mudra
Irregular Heart Palpitations	Irregular Heart Palpitations Mudra
Insomnia	Jnana Mudra + Prana Mudra

Concern	Mudras
Inner Peace/Flexibility	Matsya Mudra
Itching	Jala Mudra
Jaundice	Prithvi Mudra + Prana Mudra
Lockjaw	Akasha Mudra
Jet Lag	Akasha Mudra + Prana Mudra (50 min, in-flight)
Joint/Muscle Pain	Vayu Mudra + Prana Mudra
Kidney Problems/Stones	Kidney Mudra + Apana Mudra + Prana Mudra
Knee Joint Pain	Keela Mudra + Vayu Mudra + Jala Mudra + Prana Mudra
Lipoma	Rub Samana Mudra (5 min x 5) on the area + Surya Mudra + Apana Mudra + Prana Mudra
Liver (fatty or cirrhosis)	Shankha Mudra + Prithvi Mudra + Prana Mudra
Loose Motion	Prana Vayu Mudra + Jalodhara Nashaka Mudra
Leukoderma	Jala Mudra + Prana Mudra + place Samana Mudra on the area for 15 min
Memory	Hakini Mudra + Jnana Mudra
Menopausal issues	Surabhi Mudra + Shankha Mudra
Migraine	Maha Shirsha Mudra + Prana Mudra
Motion Sickness	Shoonya Mudra
Muscle Catch	Shoonya Vayu Mudra + Jala Mudra + Prana Mudra
Navel Disorder	Linga Mudra
Nerves issue	Prana Mudra + Shankha Mudra + Hakini Mudra + Vyana Mudra
Numbness	Shoonya Vayu Mudra + Shoonya Mudra + Prana Mudra
Obesity	Surya Mudra (30 min) + Shankha Mudra (30min) + Prana Mudra
Osteoporosis	Vayu Mudra + Akasha Mudra + Prana Mudra
Paralysis	Vyana Mudra + Shoonya Vayu Mudra (50 min each with gap in between) + Pranama Mudra (10 min) + Prana Mudra
Parkinsons	Shoonya Vayu Mudra + Jnana Mudra + Prana Mudra ((30 min + 15 min + 15 min) x 2)

Concern	Mudras
Piles	Sahaja Shankha Mudra + Prana Mudra
Pitta	Surabhi Mudra
Pleurisy	Linga Mudra + Surya Mudra + Prana Mudra
Psoriasis	Jala Mudra (50 min) + Apana Mudra (15min) + Prana Mudra (15min)
Prostate Issue	Vayu Mudra + Apana Mudra + Surabhi Mudra + Prithvi Mudra
Respiratory Issues	Pooshana Mudra + Linga Mudra + Garuda Mudra
Retinal Degeneration	Prana Mudra (20min x 2) + Samana Mudra (place on the eyes for 15 min) + Palming (rub your palms and place them on eyes for 15min x 2)
Rheumatism	Surabhi Mudra + Keela Mudra
Sciatica	Shoonya Vayu Mudra + Prana Mudra
Shivering	Linga Mudra/Surya Mudra
Sinusitis	Kubera Mudra + Prana Mudra
Slip Disc/Spine Issues	Kati Mudra + Sahaja Shankha Mudra + Prana Mudra
Sneezing	Aditi Mudra + Prana Mudra
Snoring	Simha Mudra + Lock the tongue to the upper palate + Ujjaiyi Pranayam + Adi Mudra + Udana Mudra
Speech—Stammering/ Stuttering	Udana Mudra + Shankha Mudra + Prana Mudra
Swelling	Jalodhara Nashaka Mudra
Taste Loss	Jala Mudra + Prithvi Mudra
Teeth issues	Akasha Mudra + Apana Mudra
Throat Irritation	Linga Mudra + Prithvi Surabhi Mudra
Thyroid	Shankha Mudra + Sahaja Shankha Mudra + Surya Mudra
Tonsillitis	Shankha Mudra
Tuberculosis	Linga Mudra + Surya Mudra
Tumors	Linga Mudra + Prana Mudra + place Samana Mudra on the area

Concern	Mudras
Ulcerative Colitis	Shankha Mudra + Jalodhara Nashaka Mudra + Prana Mudra
Urticaria	Prithvi Mudra + Prana Mudra (15 min x 2)
UTI	Kidney Mudra (10 min x 2) + Apana Mudra
Vayu Discomfort	Vayu Mudra + Apana Vayu Mudra
Vertigo	Shoonya Vayu Mudra (50 min) + Prana Mudra (15 min). After the problem is resolved: Akasha Mudra + Prana Mudra
Varicose Veins	Apana Vayu Mudra + place Samana Mudra on the area for 15 minutes
Weakness	Prithvi Mudra + Prana Mudra
Wealth gain	Kubera Mudra
Weight gain	Aditi Mudra
Whooping Cough	Prithvi Surabhi Mudra
Wish-fulfilment	Surabhi Mudra (minimum 21 days)
Yawning	Aditi Mudra

Bibliography

Acharya Keshav Dev Ji Maharaj. (2001). *Paravidya Gayatri (Mudra Vijnaan)* [Hindi]. Vivekananda Parishthan Parishad.

Acharya Keshav Dev and Acharya Dr. Vikramaditya. (2016). *Mudras for healing: Mudra Vigyan—A Way of Life* (1st ed.). Acharya Shri Enterprises.

Acharya Keshav Devji Maharaj and Acharya Vikramaditya. (2015) *Chamatkari Yoga Mudraayein* [in Hindi]. New Delhi: Vivekanand Pratishthan Parishad.

Aurobindo, S. (2000). *The Synthesis of Yoga*. Sri Aurobindo Ashram.

Chiplunkar, S.K. (2022). *Mudras & Health Perspectives: An Indian Approach* (29th printing). Vasantha Prakashana.

Delgado, B. J. and Bajaj, T. (2025, January). *Physiology, Lung Capacity*. In *StatPearls* [Internet]. StatPearls Publishing. https://www.ncbi.nlm.nih.gov/books/NBK541029/.

Dharanipragada, R. and Dharanipragada, D. (2021). *Sampoorna Mudra Vignan*. Dharanipragada Prakash Rao.

Himalayan Siddha Akshar. (2022). *The Science of Mudras* (Vol. 1). Clever Fox Publishing.

Hirschi, G. (2016). *Mudras: Yoga in Your Hands*. Weiser Books.

Iyengar, B.K.S. (2016). *Light on Yoga: The Classic Guide to Yoga by the World's Foremost Authority* (50th impression). HarperCollins India.

Kulkarni, A.A., and Gadgil N.D. (2022). Garbhopanishad: An Optimal Doctrine over the Embryo: A Literature Research. *Journal of Ayurvedic and Herbal Medicine, 8*(2), 88–93. https://doi.org/10.31254/jahm.2022.8206.

Menen, R. (2019). *The Healing Power of Mudras: The Yoga of the Hands* (1st ed.). V&S Publishers.

Nestor, J. (2020). *Breath: The New Science of a Lost Art*. Riverhead Books.

Priyanka, N., Gunupati, S., Nitin, V.M., Sreeshyla, H.S., and Meenakshi, S. (2019). 'Mudras'—A Traditional Boon to Dentist's Agony. *Indian Journal of Physiotherapy and Occupational Therapy – An International Journal, 13*(1), 160. https://doi.org/10.5958/0973-5674.2019.00032.7.

Rajput, M. S. (2016). The Source, Meanings and Use of "Mudra" Across Religions. *International Journal of Interdisciplinary Research in Arts and Humanities, 1*(1), 37–42. https://ijirah.dvpublication.com/uploads/667651821f3ad_7.pdf.

Saradananda, S. (2015). *Mudras for Modern Life: Boost Your Health, Re-Energize Your Life, Enhance Your Yoga and Deepen Your Meditation* (1st ed.). Watkins Media.

Saraswat, N.K. and Kumar, N. (2021). Effect of Jñāna Mudra on Anxiety Level Among Young Adults. *International Journal of Physical Education, Sports and Health, 8* (3), 31–34. https://doi.org/10.22271/kheljournal.2021.v8.i3a.2058.

Saravanan, P.S.L., Anu, S., Kanietha, P.A.S., Vijaybabu, K., and Rohit Paul. (2019). Lung-specific Yoga Mudras on Respiratory Function in Asthma Patients. *National Journal of Physiology, Pharmacy and Pharmacology, 9*(9), 878–883. https://www.njppp.com/fulltext/28-1561025032.pdf?1752017902.

Solanki, S. (2014). Vedic Vibrational Healing: First of Its Kind Unconventional Healing System—Non-Intrusive, Highly Efficacious. *Alternative & Integrative Medicine, 3*(2). https://doi.org/10.4172/2327-5162.1000156.

Sunitha, S. and Sharma, C.P. (2021). Mudra Therapy and Its Classification. *International Journal of Health Sciences and Research, 11*(1), 158–163. https://www.ijhsr.org/IJHSR_Vol.11_Issue.1_Jan2021/IJHSR16.pdf.

Swami Chinmayananda. (2000). *The Holy Geeta* (Commentary). Central Chinmaya Mission Trust.

Swami Chinmayananda. (2018). *Taittiriya Upanishad* (Kindle edition). Central Chinmaya Mission Trust.

Swami Chinmayananda. (Commentator). (2018). *Ātmabodha* (Original work by Ādi Śaṅkarācārya). Central Chinmaya Mission Trust.

Swami Maheshananda. (2009). *Shiva Samhita*. Kaivalyadhama.

Swami Muralidharan. (2010). *Kaivalyopanishad – The Key to Liberation*. Self-published.

Swami Muralidharan. (2018) *Jnaanamrutam – Nectar of Consciousness*. Self-published.

Swami Niranjanananda Saraswati. (2012). *Gheranda Samhita*. Yoga Publications Trust, Bihar School of Yoga.

Swami Satyananda Saraswati and Swami Niranjanananda Saraswati. (2013). *Mudra Vigyan: Philosophy and Practice of Yogic Gestures: From the Teachings of Swami Satyananda Saraswati and Swami Niranjanananda Saraswati*. Yoga Publications Trust.

Swami Satyananda Saraswati. (2013). *Asana Pranayama Mudra Bandha* (Golden Jubilee ed.). Yoga Publications Trust.

Swami Vivekananda. (1913). *Vedanta Philosophy: Lectures by Swami Vivekananda on Raja Yoga also Patanjali's Yoga Aphorisms, with Commentaries, and Glossary of Sanskrit Terms* (9th ed.). Baker and Taylor Company.

Swami Vivekananda. (2021). *Patanjali Yoga Sutra* (Commentary). Srishti Publishers.

Tripathi, D., Singh, R., Verma, P., Sharma, A., and Kumar, S. (2017). Effect of Yoga Hand Mudra on Cardiac and Neurological Parameters in Preventing Heart Attack. *Research Journal of Recent Sciences*, *6*(2), 16–20. https://www.isca.me/rjrs/archive/v6/i2/3.ISCA-RJRS-2017-008.pdf.

Vandali, V. and Biradar, R.B. (2018). Yoga Mudras: Benefits. *International Journal of Advances in Nursing Management*, 6(4), 324–328. https://doi.org/10.5958/2454-2652.2018.00074.4.

Yogananda, P. (1998). *Autobiography of a Yogi*. Yoganga Satsanga Society of India.

Acknowledgements

This journey with hand mudras has been deeply enriching, and I have been blessed to receive support, encouragement and inspiration from many individuals along the way. I would like to take this opportunity to express my heartfelt gratitude to a few who have played a pivotal role in shaping this path.

This book would not have been possible without the support of my son Amit and my daughter-in-law Shruti, who were among the first to believe in my work. Despite their busy schedules, they took time over the weekends to set up a website for me and have been instrumental in helping me design flyers, brochures and other promotional materials to help spread the word. Shruti continues to manage the website—regularly updating it with changes and edits to improve learner experience, often without my knowledge. Amit, meanwhile, has been actively involved in working with publishers and offering valuable insights to support the publication and release of this book. Their dedication and respect have been a source of great strength to me.

A special word of appreciation must go to my six-year-old grandson, Ved, whose spontaneous demonstrations of mudras never fail to brighten my day. His innocent enthusiasm and curiosity have been a constant source of encouragement.

I am particularly grateful to Meeta Rajani, a yoga and meditation instructor based in the UK, who has been urging me to write this book ever since she attended one of my sessions in 2023. Meeta's consistent encouragement and strong belief in the importance of this work helped bring this book into existence. I think she manifested this book more than I did. I owe its publication to her in no small measure.

My dear schoolmate and friend, Uma Rajan, a passionate teacher by profession and one of my first students, was quick to encourage me after attending my initial sessions. Her help with editing this manuscript in its early stages was invaluable, and her unwavering support has meant a great deal to me.

A special acknowledgement to Dr Priyanka Nitin, a dentist whose research paper on hand mudras—written in the context of musculoskeletal disorders among dentists—was a source of inspiration to me long before we connected. I have often quoted her research work in my courses. Hence, it was a delightful surprise to hear from her years later, expressing interest in taking my complete course.

I would like to express my gratitude to Shri Dharanipragada Prakash Rao-ji and Deepthi-ji for their invaluable guidance in hand mudras, which helped me shape and develop my course. I am also indebted to Ms Deval Delivala of GetSetUp (a platform that caters to senior citizens) for giving me opportunities to conduct hand mudra sessions on their platform. Similarly, Mr Saumyajit Roy at Emoha Elder Care has been kind enough to give me the chance to conduct programmes for seniors. Alka Jalan Foundation is yet another organisation that has given me an avenue to create awareness on hand mudras.

The people at Habuild, the Yoga Everyday community, have been consistent believers in the philosophy of mudras and have played a vital role in spreading awareness of it. Trishala Bothra and Yamini Agarwal are two among the many at Habuild who have always supported my programmes. This book also owes its fruition to the many Habuilders who have attended my courses, continually enriching my journey with their experiences and encouraging me through their appreciation.

Grateful thanks to R. Krishnan for the mudra illustrations featured in this book. His artistry has helped add a visual dimension to the book, aiding in reader comprehension.

Most importantly, I wish to thank Karthika and the wonderful team at Westland Books for believing in the book and guiding me in shaping it to its final form. Abhirami, the editor, has done a fantastic job with the book, ensuring that my thoughts reach seekers and readers with clarity and the right depth. And to Sonia, for managing the entire project end-to-end, making certain that both the most critical items as well as the smallest details are carefully considered and evaluated throughout our journey to releasing the book.

To each of these individuals—and to the many others who have supported me, whether quietly or openly—I offer my deepest gratitude. Your belief in me and in the power of hand mudras has been an enduring source of inspiration.